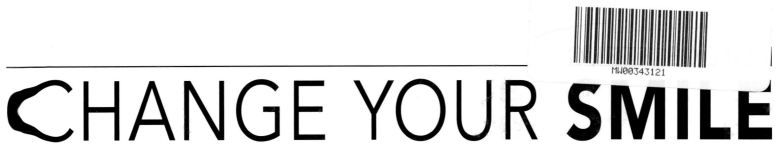

CHANGE YOUR SMILE

DISCOVER HOW A NEW SMILE CAN TRANSFORM YOUR LIFE

FOURTH EDITION

CHANGE YOUR SMILE

DISCOVER HOW A NEW SMILE CAN TRANSFORM YOUR LIFE

Ronald E. Goldstein, DDS

Clinical Professor of Oral Rehabilitation
School of Dentistry
Medical College of Georgia
Augusta, Georgia

Adjunct Clinical Professor of Prosthodontics
Henry M. Goldman School of Dental Medicine
Boston University
Boston, Massachusetts

Adjunct Professor of Restorative Dentistry
University of Texas Health Science Center
San Antonio, Texas

CONTRIBUTORS

Louis S. Belinfante, DDS
Private Practice
Oral and Maxillofacial Surgery
Dawsonville, Georgia

Farzad R. Nahai, MD
Assistant Clinical Professor
Plastic and Reconstructive Surgery
Emory University School of Medicine
Atlanta, Georgia

Foad Nahai, MD
Clinical Professor
Plastic Surgery
Emory University School of Medicine
Atlanta, Georgia

Quintessence Publishing Co, Inc

Chicago, Berlin, Tokyo, London, Paris, Milan, Barcelona,
Istanbul, Moscow, New Delhi, Prague, São Paulo, and Warsaw

Library of Congress Cataloguing-in-Publication Data

Goldstein, Ronald E.
  Change your smile : discover how a new smile can transform your life / Ronald E. Goldstein;
contributors, Louis Belinfante, Farzad R. Nahai, Foad Nahai. -- 4th ed.
      p. cm.
Includes bibliographical references.
  ISBN 978-0-86715-466-5
  1. Dentistry--Esthetic aspects. 2. Prosthodontics. I. Title.
  RK54.G63 2009
  617.6--dc22

                          2009008108

Illustrations by Zach Turner, Blue Motion Studios.

Expert beauty tips on pages 200–207 and makeup for the models on pages 203, 207, and 214 by Rhonda Barrymore, professional makeup artist and stylist and founder and president of Help Me Rhonda, Inc.

Hairstyles for the models on pages 203, 207, and 214 by Richard Davis, professional hairstylist.

Virtual hairstyle images and expert advice on pages 209–213 provided by TheHairStyler.com.

©2009 Quintessence Publishing Co, Inc

Quintessence Publishing Co Inc
4350 Chandler Drive
Hanover Park, IL 60133
www.quintpub.com

Editor: Kathryn Funk
Design: Gina Ruffolo
Production: Gina Ruffolo and Angelina Sanchez

Printed in Singapore

DEDICATION

This book is dedicated to the memory of a dentist who was the ultimate dental-patient consumer advocate. In addition to being a perfectionist and committed to excellence, he was a protector of patients' best interests.

His love of dentistry and his concern for people fueled his passion for helping others. His life and example served to inspire all who knew him. He helped me. He inspired me.

This book is dedicated, then, in loving memory to my father, Dr Irving H. Goldstein.

TABLE OF CONTENTS

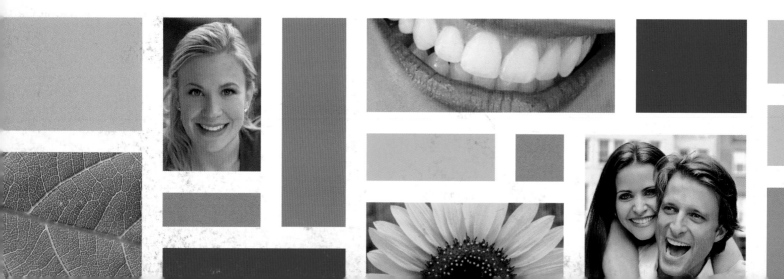

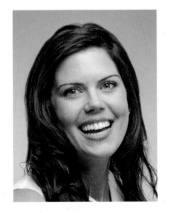
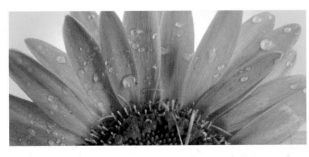
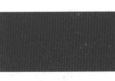
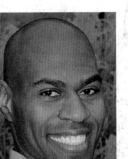

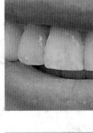

ACKNOWLEDGMENTS

A great many people have helped to make *Change Your Smile* possible. Most of them were acknowledged in the three previous editions, but certain individuals deserve recognition for making the fourth edition possible.

First and foremost, I feel fortunate to have two great clinicians in my partners and friends, David Garber and Maurice Salama, who helped me in so many ways, including reviewing many areas of the manuscript. I am very grateful to have had the help and good counsel of my mentor, Charles Pincus, of blessed memory, whom I miss dearly.

I owe a great deal of appreciation to my dentist sons, Cary and Ken, and my dentist daughter, Cathy Schwartz, who provide me with instant advice and make me very proud, as does my physician son, Rick, who also helps keep me in good health. I also want to thank my extended family—my associates who have been so helpful whenever I have called upon them, especially Henry Salama, Angie Gribble Hedlund, Brian Beaudreau, Maha El-Sayed, and Noell Craig.

So many people helped me create the esthetic results in this book that it would take too long to enumerate them. Nevertheless, this edition was aided by the talent and valuable technical skills of ceramists Pinhas Adar, Christian Coachman, Guilherme Cabral, Chris Delarm, dental technician Tony Hood, and our long-standing metalworks technician, Mark Hamilton.

This new edition was vastly improved by the splendid editorial and visual talent of Katie Funk. Thanks also go to my editorial assistant, Yhaira Arizaleta Grigsby, who handled the bulk of details necessary to bring this book to fruition. She was a tough taskmaster, but that is certainly what it takes to complete a project such as this.

A great deal of thanks goes to my entire office staff and especially to the talented dental assistants who have helped me over the years. I am indebted to our office manager Gail Cummins, accountant Chuck Gugliotta, current dental assistants Laura McDonald and Angelica Tafur, past dental assistants Maria Hernandez and Angie Moon, and particularly the unusual dedication and many other talents of Charlene Bennett. I have been privileged for more than 20 years to use the administrative abilities of Candace Paetzhold, who is the best editor and proofreader of all my writings. Our hygiene team has been of much help to me as well as to the patients. I would particularly like to thank Kim Nimmons, Gail Heyman, and the other hygienists, including Amy Bahry, Akiko Hartman, Janet Kaufman, and Cheri Robinette, who maintain the esthetic treatment of most of the patients in this book.

Some of the folks at DentalXP have aided me as well, especially Chris McGarty, Amber Vaughn, Livio Yoshinaga, and James Romeo.

Communication has always been at the core of what *Change Your Smile* is about, so I thank our treatment coordinators, Lisa Bursi, Drue Tovi, and Joy Williams, who have gone to great lengths to interpret this book's philosophy for patients. I must thank our "main man," Victor Ekworomadu, who keeps our entire office staff on track. He is the ideal employee and a real credit to mankind.

I also want to thank talented photographers Sundra Paul and Alberto Oviedo, who were helpful to me for this edition, and especially Dudu Medeiros, one of Brazil's premier photographers.

I would like to thank my terrific Medical College of Georgia team, especially Van Haywood, who has always been so gracious in sharing his material, and Dean Connie Drisko, a great faculty leader and my friend. Over the years I have gained so much knowledge and assistance from so many colleagues that I could not possibly name them all, but they know who they are, and I am eternally grateful for their dedication to the profession.

I really appreciate the contributions by Louis Belinfante and Foad and Farzad Nahai, who so beautifully show that there should be no limitation in getting the total facial look you desire. I also owe thanks to Rhonda Barrymore, Richard Davis, and the experts at TheHairStyler.com, who helped me demonstrate how makeup and hairstyles can enhance anyone's smile.

I am indebted to many others for their suggestions and especially to my family for their support and for putting up with my work habits: Amy, Jody, and Jill Goldstein; Katie, Jennie, and Steve Schwartz; and my wife, Judy, whose support, judgment, and insight continue to make this a better book.

Most of all, I never could have produced this book without the cooperation of my wonderful patients from the past 50 years (and still counting) and their willingness to share their smiles.

PREFACE

So much is new in this 25th-anniversary edition of *Change Your Smile*. The world has changed dramatically since I wrote the first edition in 1984, and so has esthetic dentistry. The treatment options for attaining the smile of your dreams are much more widely available. New materials and techniques make improving your smile less invasive and much more pleasant while providing even better results. Advancements in technology allow you not only to virtually see how great your new smile can look before any treatment begins but also to better predict how long it will last once it is completed. Technologic innovations have also enabled much more efficient communication, which means you often will have more choices based on input from your general dentist and various specialists working on your behalf—your dentist can even have an instant consultation with a specialist during your treatment!

Nevertheless, over the more than 50 years I've been practicing cosmetic dentistry, I've seen one thing remain the same—more attractive smiles dramatically improve patients' self-image. They feel better and smile more. *Change Your Smile* is designed to assure you that you don't have to go through life with a smile you don't like. You can feel better about your smile and yourself—regardless of your age, your budget, or the extent of your problem.

The critical first step is completing the smile analysis in chapter 1, which will help you determine exactly what you don't like about your smile. Do you have an underbite or overbite? Unhealthy gums? Fractured teeth? Signs of aging? You may find that the problem in your smile isn't what you thought it was or that it's not really your smile at all that needs changing. It's essential to determine this before you begin treatment, because if you address the wrong problem, you'll never be happy with the solution.

The pages that follow are filled with examples of the characteristics you might like to change in your smile. These are accompanied by the range of possible solutions. You'll learn, in a streamlined format, the benefits and potential limitations of various treatments, their costs, and how long you can expect the results to last. Not sure what a porcelain veneer is or how a crown is placed? The appendix contains simple illustrations and descriptions of all the techniques described in the book, so you'll

know exactly what is involved in any treatment you're considering. I cannot overemphasize the importance of learning as much as possible about treatment alternatives before you visit your dentist. Informed patients have a much better chance of obtaining the results they're looking for.

Use this book first to educate yourself about what you want and how you can get it, then as a tool to communicate with your dentist. Take the time to have an open conversation with your dentist and make sure your needs and expectations are fully understood and that you completely understand the treatment that is planned for you. Over the years, I've had too many patients ask me to redo their smiles because they were unhappy with the results they received elsewhere. There was no malpractice in most of these cases; instead, a lack of proper communication between the patient and the dentist led to esthetic failure.

If this describes your current situation—that is, if you've already had changes made to your smile but are still dissatisfied with your appearance—have an honest discussion with your dentist. He or she will be able to tell you if there's anything else that can be done for your smile and help you discover whether there's something else in your appearance that is actually causing your dissatisfaction. Chapter 11 presents procedures for major facial changes that can help improve your appearance and correct problems that a smile makeover cannot. If the problem is a defect that simply can't be fixed, try following the tips in chapter 12 to improve your health and beauty routines. Simple changes in your skin care, makeup, and hairstyling techniques may balance out or camouflage the problem. This is also a great chapter for those who have changed their smile but want to take the next step in improving their overall look. You won't believe the difference a few small adjustments can make in your appearance, confidence, and outlook on life.

I began writing *Change Your Smile* believing that the better educated we are about what it takes to achieve our goals and meet our needs, the more expertly we'll exercise the right to get the results we want. After you read this book, you'll know what to discuss with your dentist before you've invested your time and hard-earned money. My hope is that reading this book will give you the tools you need to better communicate with your dentist to do just that. After all, it's your smile!

1

Facing It

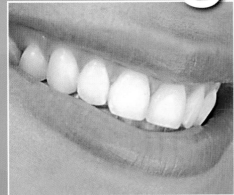

It all begins with your smile!

Your smile plays a major role in how you perceive yourself, as well as in the impressions you make on the people around you. Surveys have shown that more than any other physical feature—eyes, hair, or body—the smile is what both men and women find most attractive in other people. A charming smile can open doors and knock down barriers that stand between you and a fuller, richer life. If, on the other hand, you are dissatisfied with your smile, it may be holding you back from fully embracing life and its opportunities.

Are you ready for a new smile? Perhaps you've wondered whether straighter teeth might help you feel more confident in your professional life, or if a whiter, brighter smile might boost a dwindling social life.

If you're not completely happy with your smile, perhaps it's time to get a new one!

READY FOR A CHANGE?

If you are unhappy with your appearance, you already know it. The dilemma lies in determining where you need improvement. Many people erroneously believe that all of their facial defects reside in their smile when, in fact, their flaws may lie elsewhere. In these cases, cosmetic or oral surgery or perhaps just a new hairstyle or updated makeup, rather than dental treatment, may be more helpful (see chapters 11 and 12). Take the quiz on this page to determine if changing your smile might give you the boost you're looking for.

DO YOU NEED TO CHANGE YOUR SMILE?

Yes	No		
☐	☐	1.	Are you confident when smiling?
☐	☐	2.	Do you ever put your hand over your mouth when you smile?
☐	☐	3.	Do you photograph better from one side of your face?
☐	☐	4.	Is there someone you believe has a better smile than you?
☐	☐	5.	Do you look at models in magazines and wish your smile looked like theirs?
☐	☐	6.	When you look at your smile in the mirror, do you see any defects in your teeth or gums?
☐	☐	7.	Do you wish your teeth were whiter?
☐	☐	8.	Are you satisfied with the way your gums look?
☐	☐	9.	Do you show too many or too few teeth when you smile?
☐	☐	10.	Do you show too much or too little of your gums when you smile?
☐	☐	11.	Are your teeth too long or too short?
☐	☐	12.	Are your teeth too wide or too narrow?
☐	☐	13.	Are your teeth too square or too round?
☐	☐	14.	Do you like the way your teeth are shaped?

If you answered "no" to every question except 1, 8, and 14, you are content with your smile. Otherwise, keep reading!

1

Consider all the angles!

Keep in mind that people don't always look at you directly from the front. Defects that are minimal from one perspective may be prominent from another view. As you're performing the smile analysis, consider the angles at which people are most likely to view you. For example, if you're short, most people look at you from above. Therefore, pay particular attention to your lower teeth, especially the biting edges.

Don't overlook the details! » If you're like most people, you probably don't see what's in the back part of your mouth, but observers see it every day when you speak or laugh. Some people, such as the woman shown here, reveal most of their teeth in a wide smile. That's why it's important to evaluate every part that shows, not just those that are most apparent. (Note that the names of the teeth are provided here for reference since they're used throughout the book.)

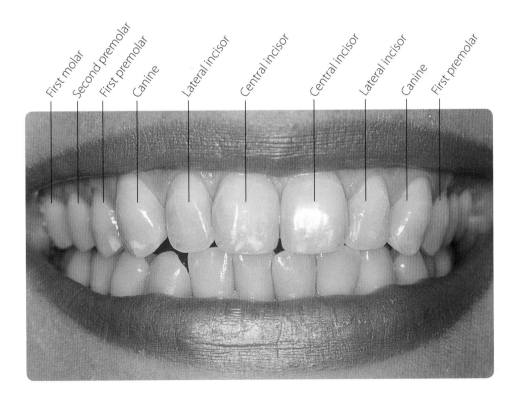

First molar | Second premolar | First premolar | Canine | Lateral incisor | Central incisor | Central incisor | Lateral incisor | Canine | First premolar

WHAT MAKES A SMILE BEAUTIFUL?

If you're not happy with your smile, or if you're curious about the possibilities of changing it, take the test on the next page. One purpose of this test is to make you aware that a smile consists of not only the front four or six teeth, but all of the teeth and gum tissue that show when you're speaking or when your lips are in your maximum smiling position. It's important to know the components of a beautiful smile so that you can discuss your particular problems with your dentist and develop a treatment plan that meets your long-term goals.

SMILE ANALYSIS

TEETH

1. In a slight smile, with teeth parted, do the tips of your teeth show?
2. Are the lengths of your central incisors in good proportion with your other front teeth?
3. Are the widths of your central incisors in good proportion with your other front teeth?
4. Do you have a space (or spaces) between your front teeth?
5. Do your front teeth stick out?
6. Are your front teeth crowded or overlapping?
7. When you smile broadly, are your teeth all the same light color?
8. If your front teeth contain tooth-colored fillings, do they match the shade of your teeth?
9. Is one of your front teeth darker than the others?
10. Are your six lower front teeth straight and even in length?
11. Are your back teeth free of stains and discolorations from unsightly restorations?
12. Do your restorations—fillings, porcelain veneers, and crowns—look natural?
13. Do any of your teeth have visible cracks, chips, or fractures?
14. Do you have any missing teeth that you have not replaced?

GUMS

15. When you smile broadly, do your gums show?
16. Are your gums red and swollen?
17. Have your gums receded from the necks of your teeth?
18. Do the curvatures of your gums create half-moon shapes around each tooth?

BREATH

19. Is your mouth free of decay and gum disease, which can cause bad breath?

FACE

20. Do your cheeks and lip area have a sunken-in appearance?
21. Does the midline of your teeth align with the midline of your face?
22. Do your teeth complement your facial shape?
23. Is the shape of your teeth appropriately masculine or feminine for your overall look?

1

WHAT DOES YOUR SMILE REVEAL?

If you've determined you're a candidate for cosmetic dentistry, it's now time to get down to specifics. Fill out the smile analysis on the facing page while looking in a close-up mirror under good lighting. On the pages that follow, find out what each of your answers can tell you about your smile.

Teeth

1 | IN A SLIGHT SMILE, WITH TEETH PARTED, DO THE TIPS OF YOUR TEETH SHOW? IF YOU SAID NO . . .

When you smile slightly and when you speak, the edges of your front teeth should show. If your upper teeth have been worn too much or if you have a low lip line (see "Read Your Lips!" later in this chapter), you may appear as if you have no teeth. **SEE CHAPTERS 8 AND 9**

This 38-year-old businesswoman was concerned with her low lip line, which made her appear as if she had no teeth. Orthodontic treatment was used to adjust her bite so her front teeth could be lengthened, then full crowns were placed on her upper front teeth.

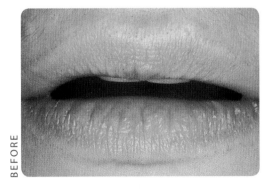

BEFORE

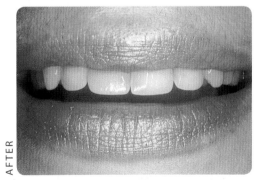

AFTER

2 | ARE THE LENGTHS OF YOUR CENTRAL INCISORS IN GOOD PROPORTION WITH YOUR OTHER FRONT TEETH? IF YOU SAID NO . . .

A *smile line* is created by drawing an imaginary line along the biting edges of the upper teeth. The most youthful and appealing smile line is one in which the two central incisors are slightly longer than the two lateral incisors. The canines should be approximately the same length as the central incisors. Your smile looks older if the teeth are all the same length (a flat smile line) or if the central incisors are shorter than the lateral incisors or canines (a reverse smile line). If the lateral incisors are too short or the central incisors are too long, the curve is too pronounced, and a "bunny look" results. **SEE CHAPTERS 8 AND 9**

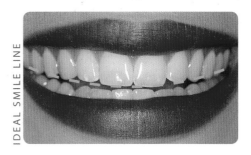

IDEAL SMILE LINE

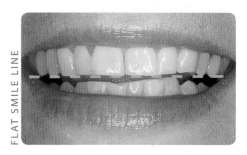

FLAT SMILE LINE

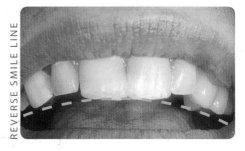

REVERSE SMILE LINE

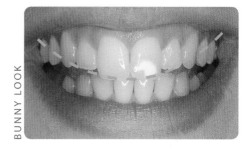

BUNNY LOOK

3 | ARE THE WIDTHS OF YOUR CENTRAL INCISORS IN GOOD PROPORTION WITH YOUR OTHER FRONT TEETH? IF YOU SAID NO . . .

Central incisors that are too wide or lateral incisors that are too narrow can make your face appear fatter. Front teeth that are too narrow may make your face appear too elongated. **SEE CHAPTER 7**

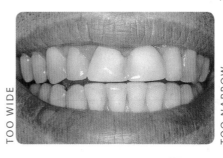

TOO WIDE

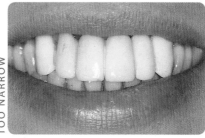

TOO NARROW

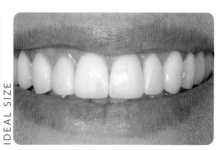

IDEAL SIZE

4 | DO YOU HAVE A SPACE (OR SPACES) BETWEEN YOUR FRONT TEETH?
IF YOU SAID YES . . .

Gaps between any of your front teeth, particularly between your central incisors, is a distraction in your smile. **SEE CHAPTER 5**

This young woman was always trying to hide the space between her teeth by placing her tongue behind it. Eighteen months of orthodontics with porcelain brackets helped create the smile of her dreams.

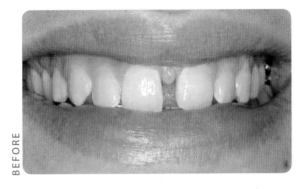

BEFORE

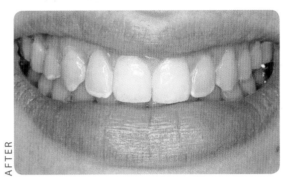

AFTER

5 | DO YOUR FRONT TEETH STICK OUT? IF YOU SAID YES . . .

Protruded teeth can cause facial deformity, not just an unappealing smile. **SEE CHAPTER 8**

This patient's teeth were loose, discolored, spaced, and so protruded that she could not even close her lips without muscle strain. Treatment consisted of periodontal gum surgery, followed by orthodontic therapy using porcelain brackets and placement of an all-ceramic fixed bridge. It took less than 2 years to transform this patient's appearance. The patient has been happily smiling ever since (and 10 years later the original bridge is still in place).

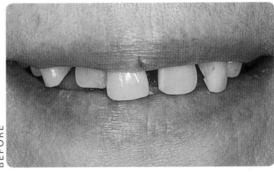

BEFORE

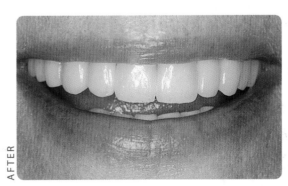

AFTER

6 | ARE YOUR FRONT TEETH CROWDED OR OVERLAPPING? IF YOU SAID YES . . .

Crowded or overlapping teeth detract from an otherwise attractive smile. Moreover, crooked teeth are difficult to clean, increasing the likelihood of gum disease, discoloration, and even tooth loss.
SEE CHAPTER 7

Crowded, discolored teeth and poorly fitting crowns made this woman embarrassed to smile. Tooth repositioning, implants, and full crowns helped to create a smile she was happy to use all the time.

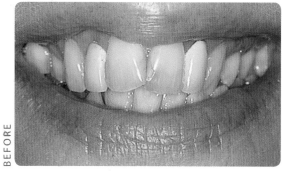
BEFORE

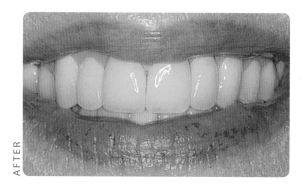
AFTER

7 | WHEN YOU SMILE BROADLY, ARE YOUR TEETH ALL THE SAME LIGHT COLOR? IF YOU SAID NO . . .

Multicolored or stained teeth are a distraction in your smile and make you look older.
SEE CHAPTERS 2 AND 9

This 20-year-old student wanted to have the color of her teeth improved for her state's Miss America competition. A series of bleaching appointments, plus minor orthodontic repositioning of her front teeth, made for a much-improved smile in only 2 months.

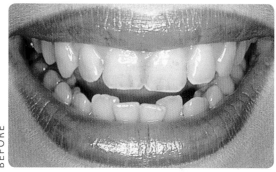
BEFORE

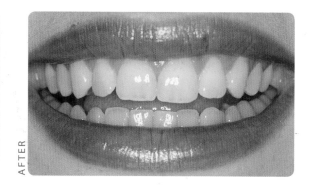
AFTER

1

8 | IF YOUR FRONT TEETH CONTAIN TOOTH-COLORED FILLINGS, DO THEY MATCH THE SHADE OF YOUR TEETH? IF YOU SAID NO . . .

Tooth-colored fillings in the front teeth, which matched perfectly when they were placed, may not look as good after a few years. Certain foods can stain these fillings, as can habits such as smoking and drinking coffee and tea. SEE CHAPTERS 2 AND 3

This 41-year-old woman was dissatisfied with her fillings, which discolored rapidly. All 12 upper and lower front teeth were bonded. Bonding teeth that have such large fillings may involve covering the entire front tooth surface. The teeth were also cosmetically contoured for a more attractive smile.

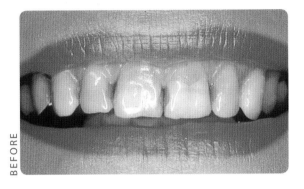
BEFORE

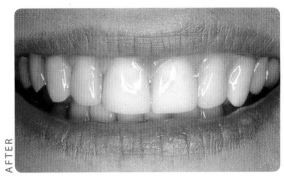
AFTER

9 | IS ONE OF YOUR FRONT TEETH DARKER THAN THE OTHERS? IF YOU SAID YES . . .

If one of your teeth is darker than the others, it may indicate that the nerve inside is injured or dead. In such cases, the nerve may require endodontic or root canal therapy to preserve the tooth before measures are taken to lighten it. SEE CHAPTER 2

This 16-year-old student had injured his front tooth. Root canal therapy was performed, then external and internal bleaching were used to lighten the tooth.

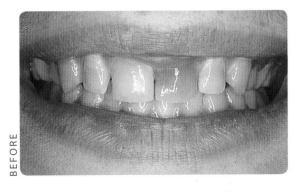
BEFORE

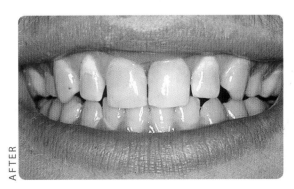
AFTER

10 | ARE YOUR SIX LOWER FRONT TEETH STRAIGHT AND EVEN IN LENGTH? IF YOU SAID NO . . .

Uneven or crooked lower teeth can be a distraction when you smile or speak. **SEE CHAPTER 7**

Crowded and uneven lower teeth were distracting in this 42-year-old businessman's smile. The teeth were reshaped in a single cosmetic contouring appointment to create the illusion of straightness.

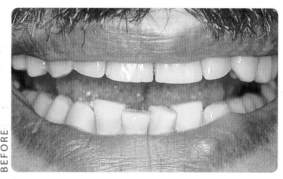
BEFORE

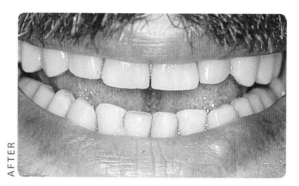
AFTER

11 | ARE YOUR BACK TEETH FREE OF STAINS AND DISCOLORATIONS FROM UNSIGHTLY RESTORATIONS? IF YOU SAID NO . . .

In a full smile, the back teeth normally show. A dark defective filling can spoil an otherwise attractive smile. Moreover, a discolored tooth may indicate decay or leakage from an old silver filling that needs to be replaced. **SEE CHAPTER 3**

This woman was unhappy with her discolored back teeth caused by her old silver fillings, which were leaking and staining the enamel. The silver fillings were replaced with tooth-colored composite fillings, which helped mask the stain. However, the fillings should have been replaced long before to avoid such dark staining and allow for a brighter tooth color.

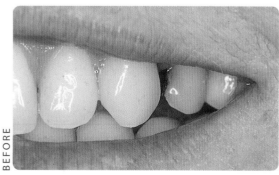
BEFORE

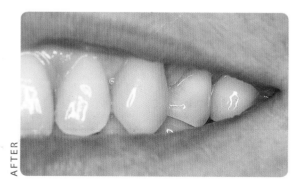
AFTER

1

12 DO YOUR RESTORATIONS—FILLINGS, PORCELAIN VENEERS, AND CROWNS— LOOK NATURAL? IF YOU SAID NO . . .

Most people want their restorations to look natural. This requires not only technical expertise but also artistry on the part of both the dentist and the laboratory technician. How much of a perfectionist are you? Rate yourself on a scale from 1 to 10. If you're a 5, a capable dentist and good technician can probably satisfy you. If, on the other hand, you are a 9 or a 10, make sure your dentist uses a top-notch or "master" ceramist. SEE THE APPENDIX

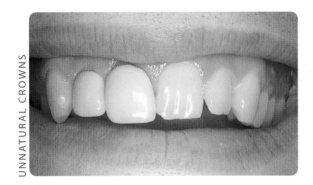

UNNATURAL CROWNS

Unnaturalness in this smile is revealed by the dark line around the two right front crowned teeth. Also, the shapes of the crowned teeth are inconsistent with the adjacent teeth. Finally, the porcelain is so opaque that it does not blend in with the color, or even the texture, of the adjacent teeth.

13 DO ANY OF YOUR TEETH HAVE VISIBLE CRACKS, CHIPS, OR FRACTURES? IF YOU SAID YES . . .

Cracks, chips, and fractures can spoil an otherwise attractive smile. Also, cracks attract staining, making them even more visible. SEE CHAPTER 4

This young man fractured his left central incisor playing soccer. In one appointment direct composite resin bonding was performed to painlessly repair the fractured tooth without any anesthetic.

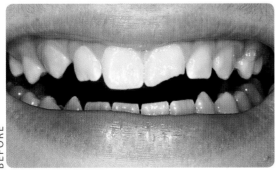

BEFORE

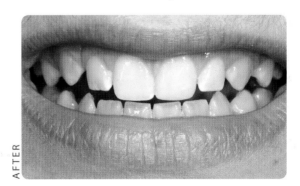

AFTER

14 | DO YOU HAVE ANY MISSING TEETH THAT YOU HAVE NOT REPLACED?
IF YOU SAID YES . . .

Missing teeth leave holes that greatly detract from your smile. Even if the missing tooth is in the back and not visible in your normal smile, it will cause the teeth to shift, eventually causing gaps in the front teeth. **SEE CHAPTER 6**

This 57-year-old artist realized that his missing teeth were a distraction in his smile. Porcelain crowns and a fixed bridge were used not only to replace the missing teeth but also to improve the color and shape of the rest of his teeth, greatly enhancing his smile.

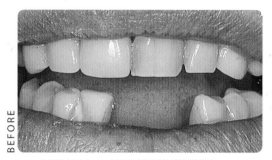
BEFORE

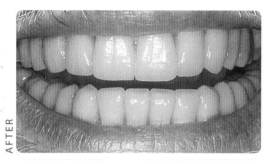
AFTER

Gums

15 | WHEN YOU SMILE BROADLY, DO YOUR GUMS SHOW? **IF YOU SAID YES . . .**

Showing the gum tissue above the teeth is referred to as a high lip line (see "Read Your Lips!" later in this chapter), and it can be sexy and attractive as long as the gum tissue is healthy looking. However, showing an excessive amount of gum tissue can ruin an otherwise attractive smile. **SEE CHAPTER 10**

This 20-year-old beauty pageant contestant was bothered by the amount of gum tissue that showed when she smiled. After cosmetic gum surgery, her teeth appeared longer and much less gum tissue showed when she smiled, giving her more self-confidence.

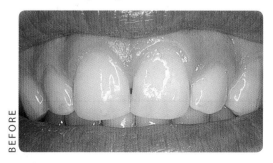
BEFORE

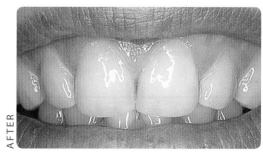
AFTER

1

16 | ARE YOUR GUMS RED AND SWOLLEN? IF YOU SAID YES . . .

Gums should be pink and well defined, not red and puffy. Dark or red gum tissue may indicate periodontal disease, an allergic reaction, or irritation from an ill-fitting restoration.
SEE CHAPTER 10

Poorly fitting crowns and veneers caused the gums of this attractive woman to become inflamed. Gum surgery, orthodontics, and new all-ceramic crowns and porcelain veneers were used not only to eliminate the gum disease but also to make this woman's smile match the rest of her pretty face.

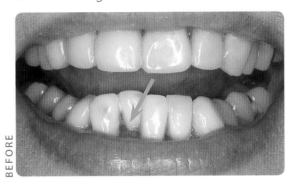

BEFORE

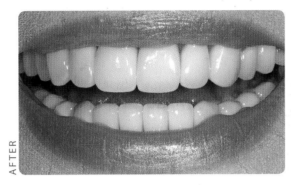

AFTER

17 | HAVE YOUR GUMS RECEDED FROM THE NECKS OF YOUR TEETH?
IF YOU SAID YES . . .

If your gums are receding or clefting, don't ignore it! This type of problem typically grows worse, eventually exposing the roots of the teeth, which, in turn, erode quickly and cause even more damage. Frequently, poor brushing habits are the culprit. **SEE CHAPTER 10**

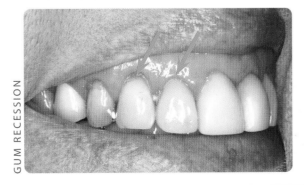

GUM RECESSION

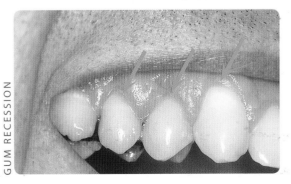

GUM RECESSION

18 | DO THE CURVATURES OF YOUR GUMS CREATE HALF-MOON SHAPES AROUND EACH TOOTH? **IF YOU SAID NO . . .**

If your gum contour is flat instead of curved, your teeth may appear too short. **SEE CHAPTER 10**

Although this woman had invested a great deal of time and money in having her teeth restored, she was terribly unhappy with the result. Note the excessive flat gum tissue around her two central incisors as well as the extremely long lateral incisors. Cosmetic gum surgery and new brighter restorations helped transform her smile.

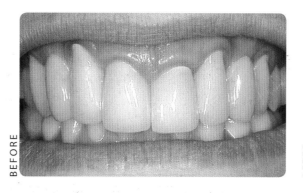
BEFORE

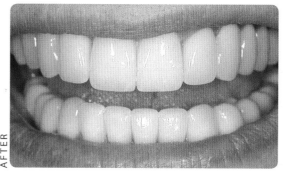
AFTER

Breath

19 | IS YOUR MOUTH FREE OF DECAY AND GUM DISEASE, WHICH CAN CAUSE BAD BREATH? **IF YOU SAID NO . . .**

No one always has pleasant breath. However, if you consistently experience bad breath—even with regular brushing and professional cleaning—it usually indicates the presence of odor-producing bacteria, generally on the back of the tongue. It can also be associated with tooth decay, gum disease, or systemic illness. **SEE CHAPTERS 3 AND 10**

1

20 | DO YOUR CHEEKS AND LIP AREA HAVE A SUNKEN-IN APPEARANCE?
IF YOU SAID YES . . .

Tooth position can affect the appearance of the whole face. The relative fullness of the cheeks is determined not only by the thickness of the tissue itself but also by the position of the underlying teeth or restorations. For example, some people with dentures look as if their lips and cheeks have collapsed. This is due to poor tooth arrangement and placement of the denture, which in turn leads to an inadequate fit.

SEE CHAPTER 6

This patient had 12-year-old dentures that did not fit him well and were falling apart. New full dentures were constructed that helped support his facial structure while improving his smile and making him look friendlier at the same time.

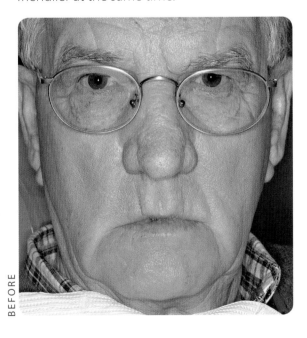
BEFORE

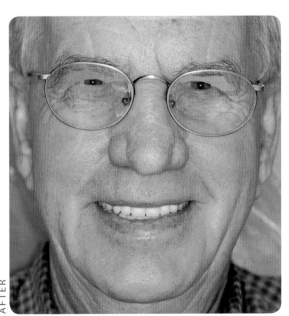
AFTER

21 DOES THE MIDLINE OF YOUR TEETH ALIGN WITH THE MIDLINE OF YOUR FACE? IF YOU SAID NO . . .

The midline of your face and its relationship to the midline of your teeth also affect the esthetics of your smile (see "Do You Have the Right Proportions?" later in this chapter). Although ideally the midline of the teeth should be in line with the midline of the face, most times it varies slightly. Facial features commonly "slant" one way or the other, so in many cases an off-center midline can be quite acceptable. What is most important is for the midline of the teeth to be parallel to the midline of the face. SEE CHAPTERS 5, 7, AND 8

This young woman had a severely deviated midline. She declined orthodontic treatment, preferring an "instant result." An effective compromise was obtained through composite resin bonding. Although the dental midline still does not match the facial midline, the smile is now more pleasing, and the midline discrepancy is hardly noticeable.

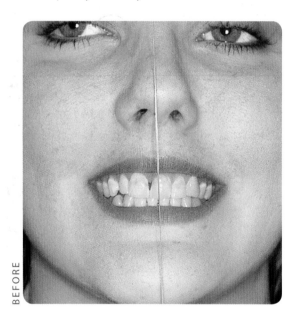

BEFORE

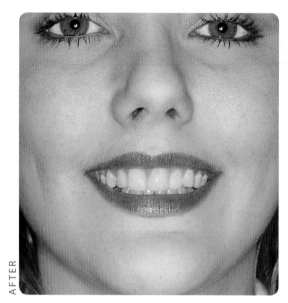

AFTER

1

22 | DO YOUR TEETH COMPLEMENT YOUR FACIAL SHAPE? IF YOU SAID NO . . .

The shapes of your teeth play a key role in your overall appearance. If you have a round face and teeth that are flat, your face will appear much wider than it really is. Likewise, long teeth will emphasize a long face, and square teeth will accentuate the squareness of a face. SEE CHAPTER 8

This pretty college senior was frustrated because her crowns had repeatedly fractured and became uncemented, so she sought a new dentist. At the consultation, her smile was analyzed, and it was determined that, in addition to her ill-fitting, short crowns, her central incisors were too wide for her face. New all-ceramic crowns, porcelain veneers, and bonding were combined to create teeth that were more proportional to each other and with her face. Note how her new hair color and style, as well as her makeup, also enhance her total facial appearance.

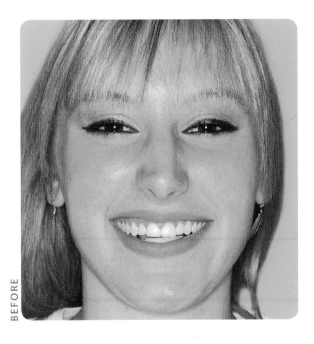
BEFORE

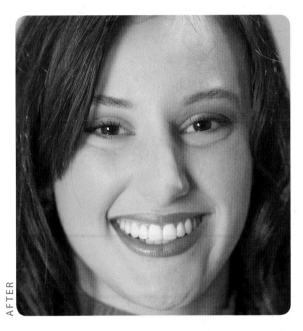
AFTER

23 | IS THE SHAPE OF YOUR TEETH APPROPRIATELY MASCULINE OR FEMININE FOR YOUR OVERALL LOOK? **IF YOU SAID NO . . .**

Generally, square teeth are considered more masculine and rounded teeth more feminine. However, there are no rules. Some women want a delicate and more rounded shape to their teeth; some prefer a bold, athletic look. Likewise, many men desire an angular "masculine" smile, while others want a softer appearance. If you aren't happy with the image your smile projects, your cosmetic dentist may be able to reshape your teeth to give them a whole new look. **SEE CHAPTER 8**

Note the subtle yet significant differences between the feminine and masculine tooth shapes.

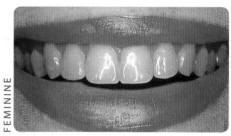
FEMININE

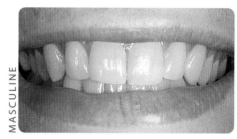
MASCULINE

Artistic cosmetic contouring can change a smile to be softer and more feminine looking.

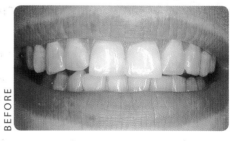
BEFORE

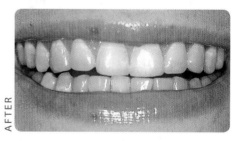
AFTER

The crowns on this 50-year-old dentist's teeth looked too feminine. They were replaced with crowns that appeared stronger and more angular to create a more masculine effect.

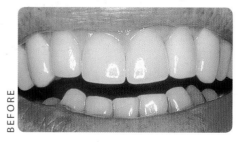
BEFORE

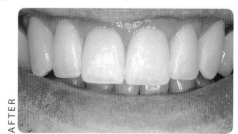
AFTER

1

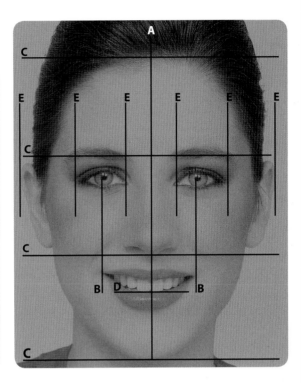

Assessing your facial symmetry » This model was chosen because her face is almost perfectly proportioned.

The face is divided into halves vertically by line A, which is the midline. It should run through the center of the nose and lips and ideally between the central incisors. Also, the pupils of the eyes should align vertically with the corners of the mouth (lines B).

Horizontally, the face should divide into approximately equal thirds at the hairline, browline, base of the nose, and tip of the chin (lines C). The distance from the base of the nose to where the lips meet (line D) should be one-third of the lower third of the face. This face also meets the ancient Greek criterion of the perfect facial width, which is five times the width of one eye (lines E).

Take a look at the pictures to the left, then examine your own face in a mirror, making sure your hair is back so you can see your complete facial outline. Are there ways in which your face is out of balance? Some asymmetry is to be expected and even desired—studies indicate that, within limits, the most appealing face is one with some sort of slight imbalance. However, being aware of your own proportions is important as you begin to make decisions about changing your appearance. Changes to your smile can make a significant difference in the overall composition of your face.

The lips are highly expressive and influence attractiveness. They play a leading role in how your face looks, affecting the prominence of other features such as your nose and chin. The relative position of your teeth in the arch of your mouth in part determines your lip position. This is important to keep in mind when you are considering cosmetic dentistry because any change in the type, size, position, or vertical or horizontal overlap of your teeth can change the look of your lips and thus your facial appearance.

Lip Line Analysis

1. When you smile normally:
   - How much of your upper teeth show?
   - How much of your lower teeth show?
2. When you smile broadly:
   - Can you see upper teeth, but not gum tissue around the teeth? (This indicates a low lip line.)
   - Can you see only the tips of the gum tissue between the teeth? (This indicates a medium lip line.)
   - Can you see a lot of the gum tissue above the upper teeth? (This indicates a high lip line.)
3. How many teeth are revealed in your widest smile?

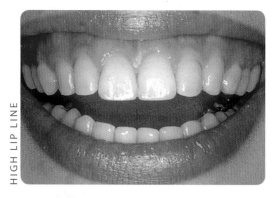

HIGH LIP LINE

What kind of lip line do you have?

- *High* lip lines expose excessive amounts of gum tissue above the upper front teeth.
- *Medium* lip lines reveal the upper front teeth and papillae (gum tissue between the teeth) up to but not including the gum tissue above the teeth.
- *Low* lip lines show no gum tissue at all and very little tooth structure.

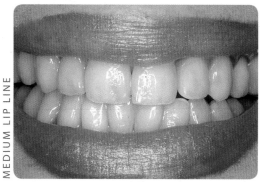

MEDIUM LIP LINE

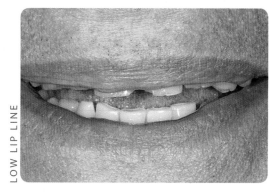

LOW LIP LINE

Lip lines can be altered » The lip line can be cosmetically modified by lengthening or shortening the teeth. This attractive young lady tried not to smile because she was embarrassed by her teeth and gums. She had a high lip line that revealed too much of her gums, and she said it affected her personality and all her relationships every day. Implants, orthodontics, bleaching, cosmetic contouring, and cosmetic gum surgery were performed to lengthen her teeth and give her a more attractive medium lip line and overall beautiful smile.

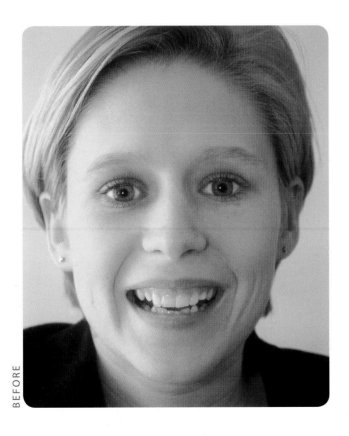

BEFORE

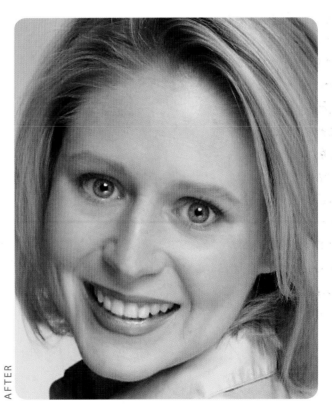

AFTER

BE CHOOSY!

For the sake of convenience, most people choose to visit a neighborhood dentist for their routine dental treatment. When seeking a cosmetic dentist, however, don't let location alone be a deciding factor. Do some research to find the very best—you'll be glad you did!

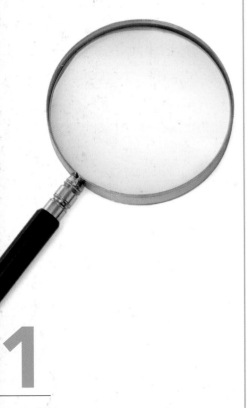

what to eXpect

ARE YOU A PERFECTIONIST?

Be honest with yourself—if you even slightly fit into this category, it is in your best interest to make this point very clear with each dentist you interview. The key is to match your artistic needs with the abilities of the dentist you select.

expert tip — Consider your dentist!

Your own dentist may be the best person to see for your cosmetic dental treatment. If you're happy with the preventive treatment your general dentist has provided, ask about his or her experience and qualifications in the area of cosmetic dentistry.

smile 101 — How do you select a good cosmetic dentist?

- Contact professionals in appearance-related fields. These include plastic surgeons, cosmetologists, hair stylists, and modeling or theatrical agencies.
- Contact local dental specialists. These include orthodontists, oral surgeons, endodontists, prosthodontists, periodontists, and dental technicians. These specialists, who are familiar with the dentists in their communities, often can provide recommendations.
- Contact the American Academy of Esthetic Dentistry (www.estheticacademy.org) or the American Academy of Cosmetic Dentistry (www.aacd.com) for cosmetic dentists in your area.
- Ask friends and business associates.
- Use the Internet to research specific areas you're interested in, but use caution (most Internet sites are not governed or overseen by state boards).
- Consult your Better Business Bureau to make sure there have been no complaints against a dentist you are considering.
- Do your homework! Don't rely on advertisements and magazines.

WHAT YOU SHOULD KNOW

HOW TO EVALUATE COSMETIC DENTISTS

▶ Once you have several referrals, evaluate each dentist's website. Compare credentials, treatment photos, educational background, and any professional teaching positions. Beware of hype!

▶ Ask for a consultation. Expect to pay a fee for the dentist's time, as well as for any x-rays, computer imaging, intraoral exams, models, photographs, or other records.

▶ Outline your expectations in a wish list before your first meeting with the dentist.

▶ Bring photographs of yourself showing what you used to look like (if you want to have your teeth restored to a previous condition) or pictures of others who have the look you want to achieve.

▶ Ask to see photographs of patients the dentist has treated with similar conditions.

▶ Don't shop for bargains. Instead, look for a dentist who will spend the time it takes to give you what you want. Otherwise, you may end up spending twice the money and time fixing mistakes.

▶ Get a wax-up. In this procedure, your dentist applies a special wax either to a cast made from your teeth or directly to your mouth to give you an idea of how the final result may look.

▶ Consider a trial smile. Removable "snap-in" teeth made of acrylic or composite resin allow you to actually "wear" your new smile before any treatment is done.

▶ Ask if the dentist is able to obtain digital images of various treatment alternatives using computer imaging.

▶ Be aware of your problems and their potential treatment alternatives before seeing the dentist by performing the smile analysis that appears earlier in this chapter.

▶ Arrive at your appointment early. You'll need time to complete forms and communicate your desires unhurriedly and in a relaxed atmosphere.

▶ Bring any x-rays or study models you have had made.

▶ Be up-front about budget restrictions. Also, bring your dental insurance information to the appointment. Although insurance typically doesn't pay for cosmetic treatment, the restorative portions of your treatment, such as crowns or bridges, may be at least partially covered.

▶ Ask if the dentist has a copy of this book. If he or she does, chances are the dentist practices many of the techniques discussed.

▶ Be willing to invest in a second or third opinion.

WHAT ABOUT FEES?

Time and expense are two factors that you must consider when seeking cosmetic dental treatment. Although it may be tempting to opt for shortcuts and bargains, remember the old saying, "You get what you pay for." The best esthetic dentistry requires a highly personalized artistic approach and thus typically is neither offered at discount prices nor covered by insurance.

what to eXpect

PAYMENT IN ADVANCE

It's customary to pay for cosmetic treatment in advance. If cash flow is a problem, try to set up the treatment in stages so you can pay as it progresses. You may also opt for doing one arch at a time, but remember that it's best to have all your porcelain restorations created at the same time for perfect shade matching. You may also consider obtaining a low-interest loan from one of the several reputable financing companies that offer them for cosmetic treatment.

smile 101 What will insurance cover?

Your insurance may cover some basic aspects of treatment, but expect to pay for most cosmetic procedures out of pocket. Begin by submitting an estimate with the proposed treatment and related costs to your carrier. Once this estimate is approved, you can begin treatment with a clear idea of your financial responsibilities. If your treatment is not required for health reasons, don't ask your dentist to falsify your records.

WHAT YOU SHOULD KNOW

YOU GET WHAT YOU PAY FOR!

When assessing fees for cosmetic dentistry:

▶ Take into account the dentist's artistic skill and experience.

▶ Ask to see photos of patients who have undergone treatment similar to what you're considering.

▶ Find out how much time the dentist is willing to spend on your treatment. Make sure that the fee reflects an adequate amount of time to satisfy your needs.

▶ Keep in mind that cosmetic dentistry is a team effort. The skill of the dentist's support staff—available dental specialists, the dental hygienist, the dental assistant, and especially the laboratory technician who fabricates your restorations—is critical.

▶ Don't base your decision solely on price. Instead, match your need for a believably natural result with what you're willing to pay.

▶ Make sure you aren't rushed during your consultation—see the fees as a long-term investment. The most important goal of any consultation is to have the entire dental team thoroughly understand your vision of the esthetic result you seek.

12 QUESTIONS TO ASK YOUR COSMETIC DENTIST

1. What are my cosmetic options?

2. What compromises may I have to accept?

3. What will the final result look like?

4. Can I see before and after photographs of patients you've treated with similar problems?

5. How long will my restorations last?

6. How well will the restorations stand up to wear?

7. What type of maintenance is required?

8. How closely will the restoration(s) match my natural teeth?

9. Will I have to change my eating habits?

10. What guarantees or warranties do I have?

11. What are my payment options?

12. Do you feel you're the best dentist to do this for me?

---

expert tip Trust your instincts!

Trust is a major factor in choosing a cosmetic dentist. Your esthetic restorations may initially appear beautiful, and your expectations may be met esthetically, but will their beauty stand the test of time? Were they designed to fit precisely and thereby not irritate the soft tissue? Because it is almost impossible for you, as the patient, to make these determinations, it is essential to find a dentist who has the training, experience, and willingness to dedicate the time needed to get exceptional, long-lasting results…in short, the dentist must earn your trust.

NOW
YOU'RE TALKING!

The secret to getting exactly the smile you want lies in open communication with your dentist. Perform the smile analysis in this chapter and read about treatment options in the other chapters of this book. Determine what you need and want, and convey this message clearly to your dentist from the beginning. Ask questions about available treatment options and make sure that you understand all of them before making any decisions. This will help you be sure your "dream smile" is attainable.

2

Stain, Stain, Go Away

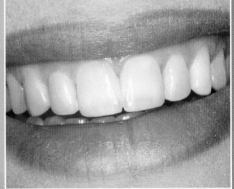

Are unsightly stains making you hide your smile?

If your teeth are stained or discolored, chances are you've gone to some lengths to achieve a whiter, brighter smile. Perhaps you've experimented with the variety of toothpastes on the market today, purchased some of the home bleaching kits sold in drugstores and supermarkets, or, in an attempt to draw attention away from your teeth, cultivated a year-round tan or accentuated your hairstyle or clothing.

Unfortunately, many of these efforts ultimately fall short. Today, however, there is no need to suffer from social embarrassment or psychological trauma because of stained or discolored teeth. Suitable cosmetic dental treatment can provide both predictable and positive long-term results.

This chapter describes the most common tooth stains and their methods of treatment.

WHY DO TEETH STAIN?

There are a number of reasons that teeth stain. Foods, beverages, and medications may discolor teeth. Smoking or forgetting to brush and floss on a regular basis may also lead to staining. In other cases, discoloration may be the result of genetics or disease.

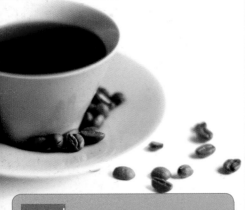

expert tip Don't chew ice!

Microcracks caused by chewing ice or other hard objects can trap stains and are difficult—or more often impossible—to clean.

2

Cut back on coffee to reduce stains » Even with frequent cleanings, stains due to drinking large amounts of coffee may rapidly return. This man's smile was greatly improved by a professional cleaning, replacement of the filling in the left central incisor, and a reduction in the amount of coffee he drank.

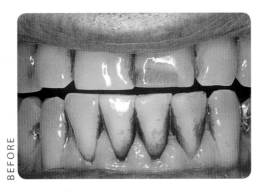

BEFORE

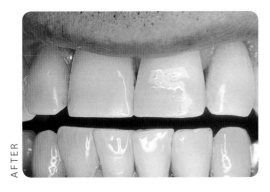

AFTER

smile 101 What stains teeth?

Stained teeth can be caused by drinking cola, coffee, and tea; consuming other stain-producing foods such as betel nuts, blueberries, or red wine; or using tobacco. These stains are called *surface stains*.

expert tip Stop staining your teeth!

- Limit the amount of coffee and tea in your daily diet.
- Avoid smoking.
- Make regular visits to your dentist for professional cleanings.
- Brush and floss regularly and properly. Some toothpastes have compounds that can help remove minor stains for a whitening effect.

Plaque can stain teeth » Plaque can build up on teeth and cause stains, referred to as *soft deposits*. This is usually the result of inadequate oral hygiene (brushing and flossing).

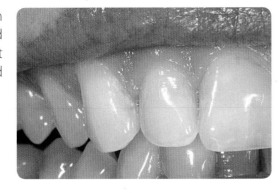

SURFACE STAINS

▶ Occur primarily between teeth and on the surfaces of crooked teeth

▶ Typically are dark brown

▶ Are caused by strong discoloring agents such as coffee, tea, and tobacco

▶ Usually can be managed with daily oral hygiene combined with regular visits to your dentist for professional cleanings

▶ May be trapped in microcracks and require a more aggressive treatment than professional cleanings alone (although bleaching can cause the microcracks to become even whiter than or a different color than the rest of the tooth)

WHAT YOU SHOULD KNOW

SOFT DEPOSITS

▶ Are caused by plaque—a sticky film that builds up on the teeth over time—or tartar (calculus)—a cement-like substance that forms when plaque is not removed

▶ Often are bacterial in origin

▶ May be the by-product of ineffective oral hygiene

▶ Can appear as dark or whitish areas around the gum line, most often on the lower front teeth

▶ Typically disappear after thorough dental scaling and polishing

Don't give up on tetracycline stains » Tetracycline stains may be yellow, dark brown, or gray. Although gray- and brown-stained teeth usually don't respond well to bleaching, multiple in-office bleaching treatments gave this patient a much whiter smile. It may take up to a year, but in many cases significant improvement in teeth with mild to moderate tetracycline stains can be achieved by bleaching using trays provided by your dentist.

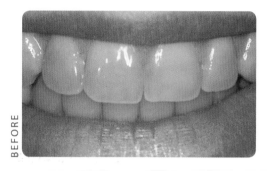
BEFORE

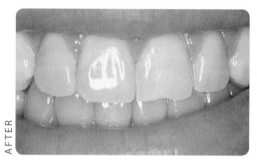
AFTER

INTRINSIC STAINS are part of the tooth structure itself. This may be a result of genetics, disease, or the use of medications such as tetracycline.

WHAT YOU SHOULD KNOW

INTRINSIC STAINS

▶ Include white splotches on the enamel surface and bands of brownish gray across the teeth

▶ May be caused by faulty hardening of the tooth before birth or the interruption of normal enamel formation by medications or disease

▶ Often appear in people who were treated with the antibiotic tetracycline before the age of 8 years or whose mothers took the drug while pregnant

▶ Can result from the use of the antibiotic minocycline

▶ May be caused by advanced decay or by old or defective silver fillings (brown or gray stains)

2

Solution 1 Polishing

is POLISHING RIGHT FOR ME?

Polishing can eliminate many minor surface stains; however, excessive or intrinsic stains may require more aggressive treatment, such as micro-abrasion. Polishing may be the best option if you:

- Have only slight surface staining
- Want a natural look rather than a very bright white smile
- Want to invest a minimum amount of time and money

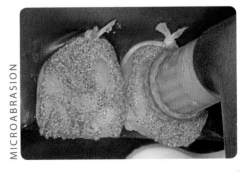

BEFORE

MICROABRASION

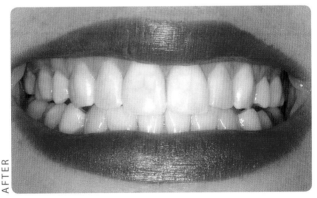

AFTER

Microabrasion » This smile was brightened using a combination of microabrasion (shown with the use of an acid polishing paste and protective rubber dam *[blue]*) and bleaching (discussed in the next section).

Solution 2 Bleaching

DOES BLEACHING WORK?

Bleaching, which uses a strong oxidizing agent to lighten the teeth, is a relatively conservative and often highly effective way to brighten your smile. Your dentist may recommend in-office or home bleaching or a combination of both, depending on the nature and severity of your stains.

is BLEACHING RIGHT FOR ME?

Bleaching is frequently used to treat mild to moderate surface and intrinsic stains but may not completely eliminate darker stains. Bleaching may be the best option if you:

- Have mild to moderate tetracycline, fluoride, or trauma-related staining
- Are on a limited budget
- Will be satisfied with a moderately brighter smile
- Are happy with the shape and proportion of your teeth
- Prefer a more conservative, noninvasive approach

Keep it simple » This 40-year-old business owner was unhappy with the color of his otherwise healthy and attractive teeth. Multiple in-office bleaching treatments achieved the color shown. It is always best to choose the least invasive option possible.

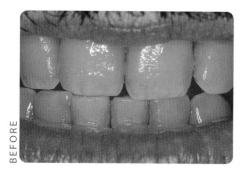
BEFORE

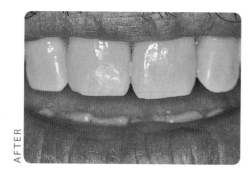
AFTER

2

expert tip Make the most of bleaching!

- If possible, sit or lie in the sunlight with your mouth open after bleaching. The tooth structure will actually absorb some of the sun's rays, which allows the bleach to continue working. Be careful, however, not to burn your skin—stay out of the midday sun, use plenty of SPF 45 or greater sunscreen, and wear loose-fitting clothing that covers your arms and legs.

- When performing home bleaching, avoid consuming citrus fruits and juices, soft drinks, and antacids. These products contain substances that when combined with the bleaching agent can slow down the tooth whitening process and cause mild irritation to the tissues in your mouth.

- Decrease your intake of refined sugars while bleaching to reduce the chance of decay. Tooth surfaces sometimes may be etched before treatment to allow greater penetration of the bleaching agent, and they can become more susceptible to bacteria. After treatment is completed, the tooth surfaces are polished to a natural and shiny luster.

Use both methods for the best results » Often a combination of professional in-office and home bleaching yields the best results. This whiter smile was achieved in 6 weeks using two in-office bleaching treatments together with home bleaching.

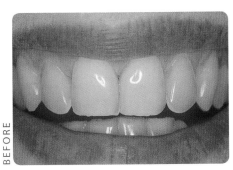

BEFORE

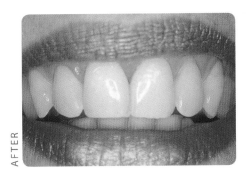

AFTER

WHAT YOU SHOULD KNOW

BLEACHING

▶ Bleaching will lighten teeth in about three out of four cases.

▶ Teeth with yellow stains are the easiest to lighten.

▶ If you bleach only your upper teeth first, you can monitor your progress by comparing the lightened upper teeth to the stained lower teeth.

▶ If you have both crowns and natural teeth that you want lightened, be sure to bleach the teeth first. Your dentist then can match a new crown to your lighter natural teeth.

▶ Bleaching may cause some discomfort in children; therefore, it's often better to postpone bleaching until they're older.

▶ Don't ask for a local anesthetic during in-office bleaching. It's important to be aware of any sensitivity.

what to eXpect

IN-OFFICE BLEACHING

The methods used for bleaching teeth in the office depend on whether your teeth have undergone root canal therapy. Teeth that have received this treatment are termed *nonvital* because they've had the nerves removed.

If you've never had root canal therapy…

- Your dentist will isolate the teeth being treated, which protects the gums from discomfort and irritation.
- The outside of the teeth will be coated with a chemical solution and may be exposed to heat and/or a special light for 20 to 30 minutes.

If you have received root canal therapy…

- The root canal will be reopened, a bleaching solution placed inside, and the canal resealed with a temporary filling.
- Heat and/or light can be used at the dental office to accelerate the whitening process.
- The bleaching agent will be removed when you and your dentist determine that you've achieved the desired tooth shade.

Leave the office with a gorgeous new smile » In-office bleaching treatments removed the dark stains from the lower portions of this woman's two front teeth. She is pleased with her new smile, which now radiates from every view.

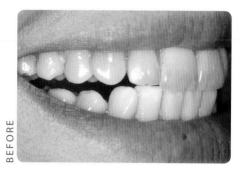

BEFORE

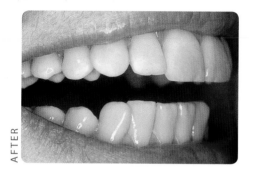

AFTER

Brighten your teeth from the inside out » The dark front tooth, which had been previously treated with root canal therapy, was first treated with a single in-office bleaching to the outside of the tooth. Then a bleaching solution was placed into the empty pulp chamber to bleach the tooth from within. After 1 week, the natural tooth color was restored, at which time the solution was removed and a tooth-colored filling placed.

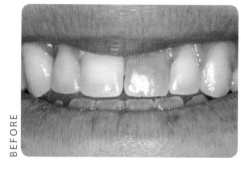

BEFORE

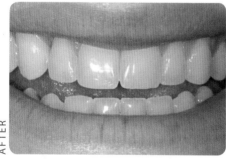

AFTER

expert tip

Let your dentist do the bleaching!

In-office bleaching is often the most effective way of lightening your teeth because the agents are stronger and the procedures more controlled compared with using over-the-counter bleaching kits.

Bring bleaching home with you!

Your dentist can provide you with a customized professional bleaching kit you can use at home. This is often called home bleaching, matrix bleaching, or nightguard vital bleaching. In addition, over-the-counter bleaching kits can be great tools for maintaining or touching up the new smile you achieved using professional bleaching. Your dentist can help you choose the best product to fit your needs.

Bleach at home for great results » This woman's tetracycline stains were removed after 9 months of nightguard vital bleaching. (Courtesy of Dr Van B. Haywood, Augusta, GA.)

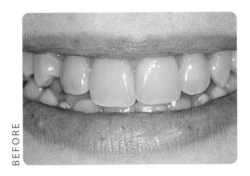

BEFORE

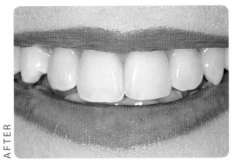

AFTER

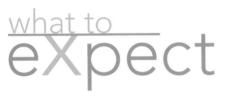

what to eXpect

PROFESSIONAL HOME BLEACHING

- You will place one drop of the bleaching gel per tooth in the plastic tray.

- The tray will fit over your teeth and typically will need to be kept in place for 1 to 3 hours each day, depending on your schedule and your dentist's recommendations. However, there are some professional bleaching gels that require fewer than 5 minutes of application daily.

WHAT YOU SHOULD KNOW

PROFESSIONAL HOME BLEACHING

▶ Although the average treatment time is about 4 to 6 weeks, you may notice results after just a few days.

▶ If you have decay, be sure to have your teeth treated prior to bleaching.

▶ Patients who are not good candidates for in-office bleaching because of tooth sensitivity, time restrictions, or financial considerations can often be helped with home bleaching.

▶ For most patients, a combination of home and in-office bleaching yields the best results.

▶ You may need a "touch-up" bleaching session every 6 to 12 months.

▶ Do not use any home bleaching product if you are pregnant or nursing a baby.

▶ Home bleaching can have adverse side effects, including tooth sensitivity, a burning sensation in the gums, soft tissue sores or ulcers, or a sore throat from swallowing the bleach.

Solution 3 Bonding

WHAT IS BONDING?

Bonding involves the application of composite resin to the existing tooth. The bonding technique is used frequently as a conservative method of covering stains.

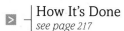 How It's Done
see page 217

is BONDING RIGHT FOR ME?

Bonding can mask many types of stains to create a natural-looking and attractive smile. However, bonded teeth tend to stain easily and require periodic repair. Bonding may be the best option if you:

- Have white or brown spots or staining due to excessive wear or silver fillings
- Are not a heavy smoker or coffee drinker
- Are willing to take extra care of your new smile
- Want a less expensive and less invasive option (compared with porcelain veneers or crowns)

Bonding for better shade and shape » This 40-year-old real estate agent was embarrassed to smile because of his discolored and worn teeth. Composite resin bonding was done in one appointment to create a much more attractive smile. In addition, cosmetic contouring was performed on the lower front teeth to make them appear straighter.

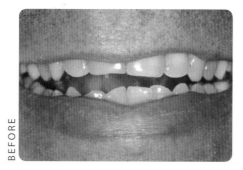

BEFORE

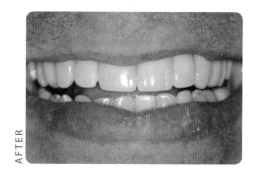

AFTER

Fillings can stain too » This 41-year-old woman was dissatisfied with her fillings, which had discolored rapidly. Bonding teeth that have large fillings often involves covering the entire front tooth surface. If the teeth were merely refilled, it would only take a short time before the junction of the filling and enamel became a site of new discoloration. To achieve this new attractive smile, her upper and lower front teeth were bonded and cosmetically contoured.

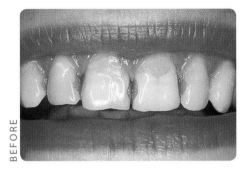

BEFORE

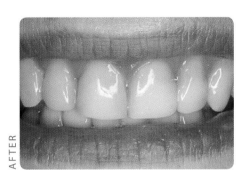

AFTER

Simple solution for tetracycline stains » This young woman's teeth had been discolored by use of the antibiotic tetracycline. With composite resin bonding, a one-day appointment was all it took to create a more radiant smile.

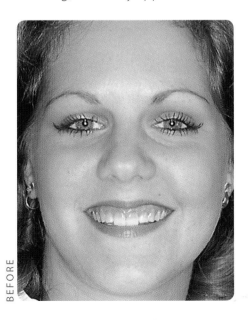

BEFORE

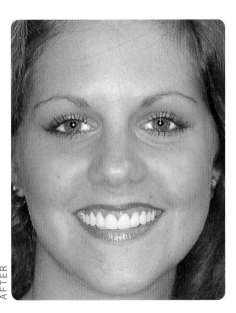

AFTER

TAKE CARE OF YOUR BONDED TEETH

- Do not chew ice or bite your finger-nails.
- Brush regularly—plaque must be removed daily.
- Floss teeth at least once daily, but pull floss out horizontally, not vertically.
- Have your teeth cleaned at least three or four times yearly. Be certain that the hygienist avoids using ultrasonic scaling or air abrasives on the bonded teeth.
- If you clench or grind your teeth at night, use a nightguard.
- Minimize your consumption of stain-causing food and drink, such as coffee, tea, and colas, as well as sugar, which can cause stains and premature loss of the restoration.
- Don't smoke.
- Avoid biting into hard foods, such as ribs, hard candy, apples, carrots, and nuts. Cut your food into small pieces and use your back teeth to chew.
- Never try "getting used to" a new bite. Go on a soft diet for the first 24 hours after treatment, then carefully assess your bite. If it's not perfect, return to your dentist to have it adjusted.
- Take daily multivitamins for 1 month before and after treatment if gum tissue is inflamed.

Solution 4 Porcelain Veneers

WHAT'S TO LOVE ABOUT PORCELAIN VENEERS?

One of the most exciting techniques in cosmetic dentistry today involves bonding a thin laminated veneer made of porcelain to the etched enamel tooth surface. Its primary advantages are the beauty and durability of the material. Because porcelain doesn't stain like composite resin, it remains attractive for a much longer period of time. In addition, gum tissues tolerate porcelain well.

> **How It's Done**
> *see pages 218–219*

are PORCELAIN VENEERS RIGHT FOR ME?

Although porcelain veneers provide excellent esthetic results, a primary disadvantage is that the laminate may chip. Porcelain veneers may be the best option if you:

- Want a significant change in the color of your teeth
- Are willing to undergo slightly more invasive and time-consuming dental procedures
- Can afford the higher cost of treatment
- Want highly esthetic results with reduced potential for staining
- Have a favorable bite

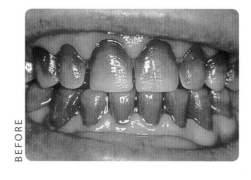

BEFORE

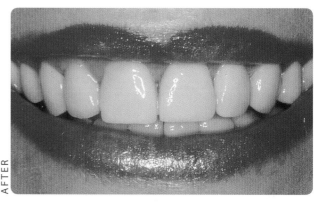

AFTER

Some stains are too dark to bleach » Tetracycline use caused severe staining on this professional dancer's teeth. Twenty porcelain veneers were placed to successfully mask the staining. To create a natural look, it is important to restore all teeth that show in your widest smile.

Subtract years from your smile » This woman felt her stained teeth were aging her smile. A much lighter color was achieved by laminating the fronts of the teeth with porcelain. This conservative approach saves enamel, thereby helping to preserve the health of the teeth as well.

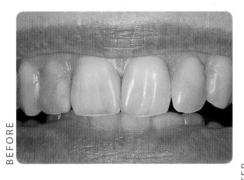

BEFORE

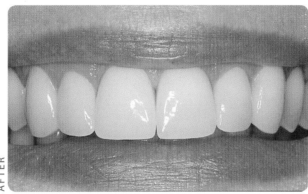

AFTER

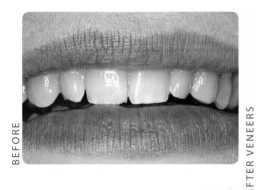

BEFORE

AFTER BLEACHING

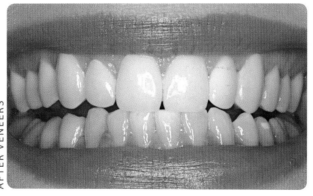

AFTER VENEERS

Stains: An unwanted side effect » This patient had a beautiful smile before she began taking minocycline, an antibiotic often prescribed to treat acne. Although her teeth got somewhat whiter with in-office and home bleaching, it took porcelain veneers to satisfy the patient's desire to restore her great smile.

Solution 5 Crowns

WANT MORE THAN JUST WHITER TEETH?

Crowns generally are not recommended for stained but otherwise healthy teeth since placing crowns requires so much natural tooth structure to be removed. However, crowns may be indicated for teeth with severe discolorations or for moderately discolored teeth that have additional esthetic and/or functional problems.

> How It's Done
> *see pages 220–225*

are CROWNS RIGHT FOR ME?

Placing crowns is a more costly and time-consuming option compared with the other solutions presented in this chapter. However, when done correctly, it can produce near-perfect esthetic results. Crowns may be the best option if you:

- Have many large defective fillings
- Want the most esthetic and longest-lasting results
- Are looking for a complete smile makeover, including improvement in the shape of your teeth
- Have discolored teeth that also need some realignment or straightening but do not desire orthodontic treatment

Take years off your smile » This retired executive became aware that his smile made him look older than he felt. Since this patient had many old restorations as well as severe microcracks in his teeth, all-ceramic crowns were chosen to provide the longest life expectancy while also improving his bite. Now he looks as young as he feels.

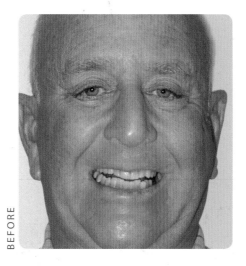
BEFORE

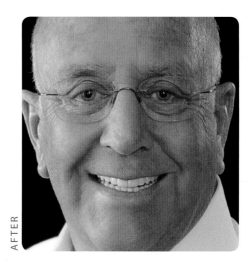
AFTER

2

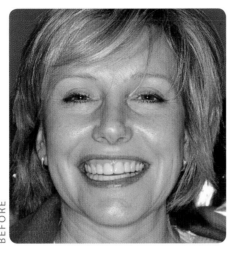

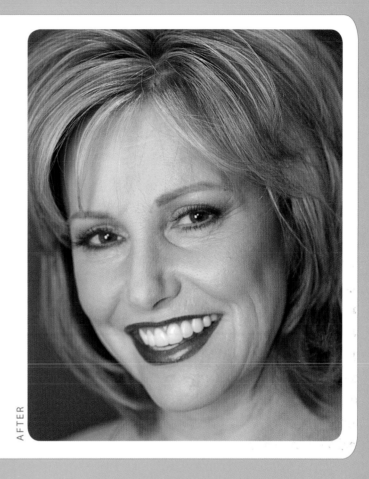

BEFORE

AFTER

Don't settle for yellow crowns »
Old yellow crowns and an irregular arch alignment were ruining the smile of this vivacious lady. Cosmetic gum surgery and new brighter all-ceramic crowns in much better alignment helped transform her smile. Now her smile is as attractive as the rest of her face.

Make your smile work for you »
This attractive woman felt her discolored teeth were making her look much older than she was. It took ten all-ceramic crowns, plus cosmetic contouring, to create a brighter and younger-looking smile. Now, rather than detracting from her beauty, this patient's smile enhances her face.

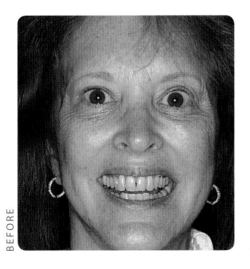

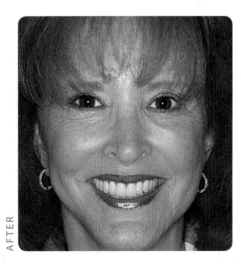

BEFORE

AFTER

WHICH SOLUTION IS BEST FOR **YOU?**

	POLISHING	BLEACHING
TREATMENT TIME	Usually a 15- to 30-min appointment	*In-office:* 1–3 treatments as needed, about 30–90 min each *Home:* Daily for 1–12 mo, depending on stain severity
MAINTENANCE	Have a professional cleaning 4–6 times per year	• Brush thoroughly after meals to remove plaque. • Avoid smoking and stain-causing foods (eg, coffee and tea). • Have a professional cleaning 3–4 times per year.
RESULTS	Surface stains easily removed	Deep yellow stains can be considerably lightened; brown and gray stains are much more difficult to bleach.
TREATMENT LONGEVITY*	Usually 2–6 mo	Indefinite, although annual touch-ups may be required
COST†	$150 to $300 depending on who does the treatment (hygienist or dentist)	$250 to $1,000 per treatment
ADVANTAGES	• Least invasive procedure • Can be least expensive option • Painless • Safe • No tooth reduction required	• Safe • Usually painless to adults • No tooth reduction required • No anesthetic required • Less expensive than many other options
DISADVANTAGES	• May not remove stains enough to please you	• Natural tooth color may not be restored. • Can cause discomfort if large tooth pulp present. • Only 85% effective in selected cases. • Extended treatment time may be necessary. • May not achieve the whiteness you desire.

*This estimate is based on the author's clinical experience combined with three university research studies and insurance company estimates. Your own experience could be different, depending on many factors, only some of which you and your dentist can control.

†Fees will vary from dentist to dentist based on the difficulty of the procedure, patient problems, patient dental and medical history, expectations, and dentist qualifications, including technical and artistic expertise.

‡Expect to pay extra for esthetic temporaries.

BONDING	PORCELAIN VENEERS	CROWNS
1 office visit	2 office visits, 1–4 hours each	Usually 2 office visits of 1–4 hours each for up to 4 teeth (more time needed for additional teeth, esthetic temporaries, or more extensive treatment)
• Have a professional cleaning 3–4 times per year. • Avoid use of ultrasonic scalers and air abrasives during hygiene office visits. • Avoid biting down with front teeth, especially on hard foods. • See dentist for polishing or repair as necessary.	• Have a professional cleaning 3–4 times per year. • Avoid use of ultrasonic scalers and air abrasives during hygiene office visits. • Take special care when biting into or chewing hard foods. • See dentist for resealing of margins as needed.	• Avoid biting down on hard foods and ice. • Reduce intake of refined sugars. • Have a professional cleaning at least 3–4 times per year and yearly fluoride treatments. • Ask your dentist to recommend a fluoride toothpaste and mouthwash for home use. • Floss at least once daily.
Immediate masking of stains	Glazed, natural appearance and effective masking of stains	Can achieve the best results in tooth shade, shape, and size
3–8 years; may need repair or replacement more frequently	5–12 years	6–15 years (directly related to fracture, problems with tissues, and decay)
$250 to $1,750 per tooth	$950 to $3,500 per tooth[‡]	$850 to $3,500 per tooth[‡]
• Painless • Results obtained in 1 appointment • Little or no tooth reduction required • Generally no anesthetic required • Less expensive than porcelain veneers or crowns • Easy to repair	• Less chipping than bonding. • Extremely good bond to enamel. • Minimal staining and loss of color or luster. • Less tooth reduction required than crowning. • Lasts longer than bonding. • Gum tissue tolerates porcelain well. • Generally no anesthetic required. • Color change is possible.	• Teeth can be lightened to any shade. • The dentist can improve shape of teeth. • Some realignment or straightening of teeth is possible. • Last longer than any other restoration.
• Can chip or stain. • Has a limited esthetic life. • May not cover dark stains well. • May involve minor tooth reduction to remove some of the stains. • Gum irritation may occur if margins are imperfect.	• More expensive than bonding. • Difficult to repair if the veneer cracks or chips. • Irreversible if much enamel is removed. • Staining may occur between teeth, depending on how the veneer is prepared. • Margins may "wash out" and require repair.	• Can fracture. • Require an anesthetic. • Tooth form is altered (most of the tooth enamel is removed). • Unsightly line may appear at junction between tooth and crown if tissue shrinkage occurs. • Much more expensive than bonding.

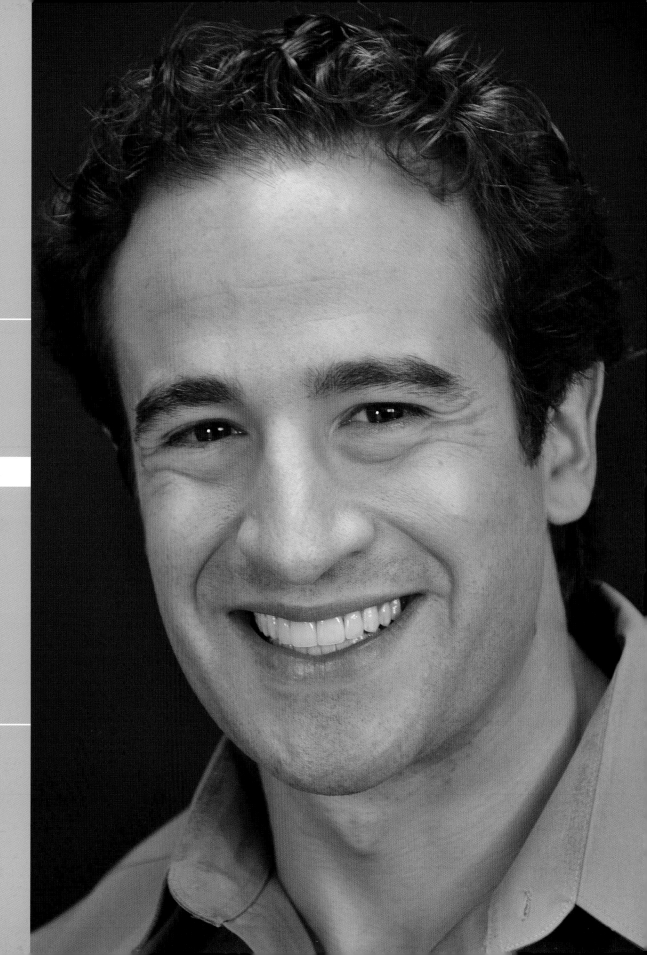

3

FIND OUT . . .

Coming Clean

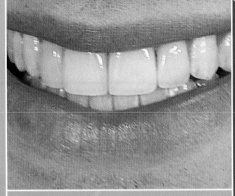

Spruce up your smile by eliminating decay and old silver fillings.

Decay and old or defective silver fillings often cause the teeth to become discolored and unsightly. If you have this problem, several alternatives are available. However, before the best option can be chosen, all decayed tooth and/or old filling material must be removed.

This chapter presents options for restoring decayed teeth and replacing old fillings, with rationales for each. It is important to note, however, that sometimes even after an old filling is replaced, stains are left behind on the remaining tooth structure. Such staining most likely will require masking using bonding, porcelain veneers, or crowns.

WHY
DO TEETH DECAY?

Decay of tooth enamel is caused by certain types of acid-producing bacteria that attack the tooth enamel located on the tooth's surface. Once the enamel surface is broken, the tooth can no longer repair itself. Continuing decay undermines the inner tooth and attacks the nerve, causing toothache.

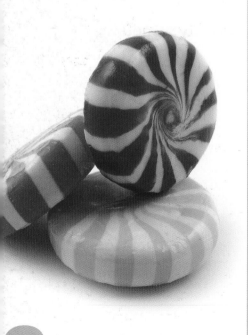

smile 101 — What is a cavity?

Caries is a term commonly used for tooth decay. The earliest sign of a new caries lesion may be the appearance of a chalky white spot on the surface of the tooth, indicating an area of demineralization of enamel. As the lesion continues to break down the enamel, it may turn brown and will eventually turn into a cavitation (cavity). Once a cavitation forms, the lost tooth structure cannot be regenerated. Your dentist will remove the decay using a dental drill, air abrasion, or laser. This creates a prepared cavity, which will receive and retain a restoration, usually a tooth-colored filling.

expert tip — Out with the old!

Dental fillings replace tooth structure lost to decay. Dental fillings may last many years; however, bacteria or stress from clenching or grinding may eventually cause the seal between the tooth and the filling to break down. Food particles and bacteria can access the area between the tooth and the filling, eventually destroying your healthy tooth structure. During regular dental examinations your dentist should determine whether existing fillings are intact. If a seal is worn, cracked, or leaking, it may need to be replaced or repaired.

expert tip — Healthy teeth are beautiful teeth!

You can help prevent tooth decay by taking steps to limit bacteria on your teeth:

- **Brush and floss daily.** Consult your dentist for his or her recommendations for the best toothpaste and type of toothbrush for your mouth.

- **Eat healthy foods**, especially whole grains, vegetables, fruits, and foods that are low in saturated fat and sodium.

- **Avoid foods that contain a lot of sugar**, especially sticky, sweet foods such as caramels and hard candies since the longer sugar stays in contact with your teeth, the more damage it can do.

3

WHAT YOU SHOULD KNOW

SILVER FILLINGS

can ruin even the most
beautiful smile. It is
worth the cost to opt for
a more esthetic solution.

Gray matters » If a silver amalgam filling
corrodes, the mercury or tin can leak into the
inner walls of the tooth, changing its color
and creating an unwanted distraction when
you are smiling or talking.

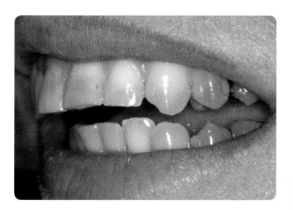

SILVER AMALGAM

Decay can be treated with a silver amalgam filling. Although simple
and cost-effective, most patients feel this is not a very esthetic
solution, as the silver often shows when you are talking or
laughing, even in back teeth. For this reason, silver amalgam fillings
are not a featured solution in this book.

ADVANTAGES

- ▶ Completed in
  one appointment

- ▶ Least costly option for
  restoring decayed teeth

- ▶ Predictable and long-
  lasting results

DISADVANTAGES

- ▶ Visibility of metal

- ▶ Tooth discoloration possible

- ▶ Can corrode

- ▶ Contains mercury

- ▶ Not sealed to tooth

- ▶ Non-insulating
  (conducts heat and cold)

- ▶ Less suited for large cavities
  (covering a cusp)

Solution 1 Composite Filling

WHY COMPOSITE?

If the cavity left by the removed decay or filling isn't too large, composite resin can provide a cosmetically appealing filling alternative, particularly in lower back teeth that show when you smile or laugh.

is TOOTH-COLORED COMPOSITE RIGHT FOR ME?

Tooth-colored composite resin offers a conservative but esthetic approach to filling cavities. A composite filling may be the best option if you:

- Are getting a small filling in an area that is visible during smiling or talking
- Want to keep cost and time of treatment to a minimum
- Are willing to accept an option with reduced longevity and resistance to wear and staining
- Want to keep as much of your existing tooth structure as possible

Take out the gray » This woman was concerned about the silver filling in her lateral incisor (*arrow*), which was causing a noticeable discoloration. Replacement of the defective amalgam filling with composite resin helped to restore proper color to the tooth. It is generally advisable to use tooth-colored filling materials in the front teeth when possible.

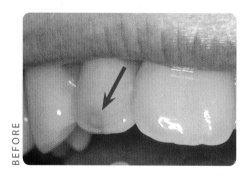

BEFORE

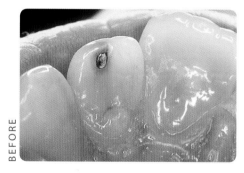

BEFORE

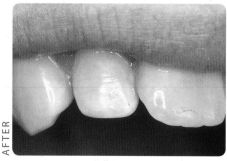

AFTER

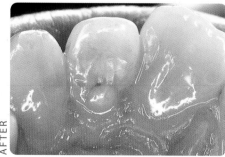

AFTER

3

Solution 2 Inlays or Onlays

are INLAYS OR ONLAYS RIGHT FOR ME?

Inlays and onlays are durable alternatives for restoring large cavities. An inlay or onlay may be the best option if you:

- Don't mind spending more time and money to get a long-lasting result
- Have a large cavity to be filled
- Want to avoid staining

What are your old fillings saying about you? » Silver and gold restorations can show when you speak and smile widely. See the difference for this patient when composite resin inlays and onlays were placed on the right side compared to the old silver and gold restorations on the left side.

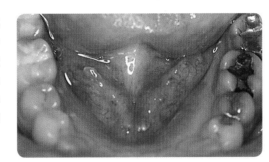

WHAT ARE INLAYS AND ONLAYS?

Inlays and onlays are particular types of fillings made of composite resin, porcelain, or gold. An inlay is custom-made to fit the prepared cavity, while an onlay covers the entire chewing surface of the tooth. The primary disadvantage of inlays and onlays is their higher cost relative to traditional composite and amalgam fillings.

WHAT YOU SHOULD KNOW

GOLD
Gold doesn't discolor or stain the teeth and has a longer life expectancy than silver. It can be placed esthetically into upper back teeth where it doesn't show; however, it shouldn't be placed opposite porcelain, because porcelain tends to wear gold rapidly during chewing.

PORCELAIN
Research shows that bonded porcelain inlays and onlays can equal the strength of natural teeth, making them particularly attractive choices when both esthetics and strength are required. However, extra stress can fracture porcelain just as it can natural teeth.

COMPOSITE RESIN
Although not as long lasting as gold or porcelain, composite resin inlays and onlays are an esthetic and less expensive option.

Solution 3 Porcelain Veneers

WHY CHOOSE PORCELAIN?

Porcelain veneers are an excellent option for front teeth with stained or defective fillings. Porcelain does not stain and is a more long-lasting solution, making it a good choice, especially if you want to improve the shape of your teeth or make other changes to your smile.

> **How It's Done**
> *see pages 218–219*

expert tip **Bleach first!**

If you would like your teeth to be lighter, be sure to bleach them before any restorations are placed so your dentist can match the crowns or veneers to the lighter shade.

are PORCELAIN VENEERS RIGHT FOR ME?

Porcelain veneers are a highly esthetic option for restoring front teeth. However, they are more expensive than composite fillings and require reduction of natural tooth structure. Porcelain veneers may be the best option if you:

- Have front teeth with extensive decay or old fillings that are discolored
- Would like to close minor spaces between your front teeth
- Are frustrated by fillings that continue to stain or are too visible
- Want a smile makeover that will improve tooth shape and brighten tooth color

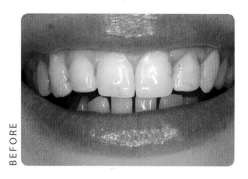
BEFORE

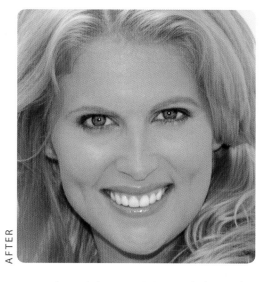
AFTER

Go places with a brighter smile » This actress and model was concerned about the color of her teeth and her stained fillings as well as the spaces between her lower front teeth. Ten porcelain veneers were placed to brighten and improve the shape of her smile. A more confident smile is an obvious advantage to someone in the modeling and acting fields, but it is also a major asset in any profession.

3

Crowns

are CROWNS RIGHT FOR ME?

Crowns can produce near-perfect esthetic results. However, both the cost and the number of office visits required may make this treatment prohibitive for some patients. Crowns may be the best option if you:

- Have extensive decay and/or severe staining following the removal of a large filling
- Are looking for the most beautiful, long-lasting result possible
- Are willing to undergo more extensive treatment and incur higher costs
- Have additional esthetic or functional concerns that can be best addressed with crowns

Take it a step further with crowns » Discolored old fillings, combined with tooth wear and a high lip line, deprived this woman of an attractive smile. Although the extent of decay and staining alone did not require crowns, her additional cosmetic concerns were best addressed using this long-lasting and esthetic solution. Cosmetic gum surgery was performed to raise her gum line, then 12 all-ceramic crowns were constructed to transform her smile. By lengthening the front teeth and matching the curve of the lower lip, a brighter and younger-looking smile was created, enhancing the beauty of her face.

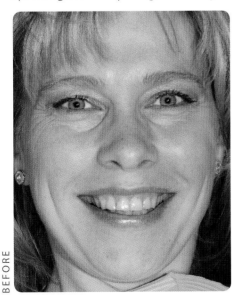

BEFORE

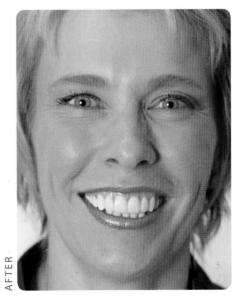

AFTER

WHEN IS A CROWN REQUIRED?

Crowns represent a long-lasting treatment alternative involving reducing the tooth and covering the remainder with a custom-made restoration. Although it's always preferable to preserve the structure of the natural tooth, if a tooth is severely decayed or stained following the removal of a large filling, placing a crown may be the best option.

> **How It's Done**
> *see pages 220–225*

THREE POPULAR WAYS TEETH ARE REBUILT

COMPOSITE FILLING

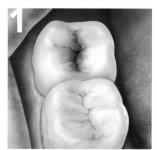

1 The second molar is decayed.

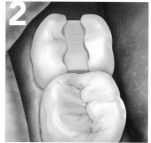

2 The decayed portion is removed, and the tooth is prepared to receive a posterior composite resin filling.

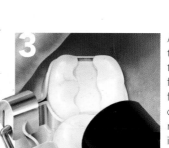

3 A band is placed temporarily around the tooth to help form the new filling. Tooth-colored composite resin is condensed in layers, each hardened with a high-intensity light.

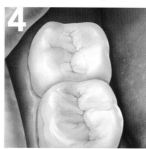

4 The final tooth-colored filling blends in naturally with the other teeth.

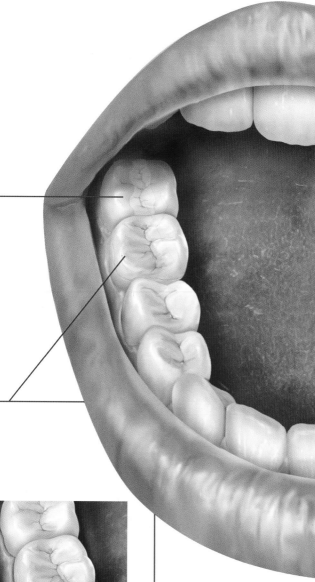

PORCELAIN ONLAY

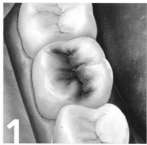

1 This first molar has a large decay area.

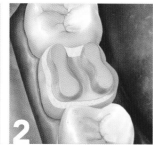

2 Because of extensive decay, much of the tooth is reduced. An impression is made, and a porcelain onlay is constructed.

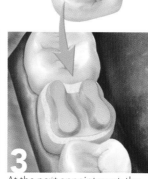

3 At the next appointment, the etched porcelain onlay is fit and bonded to the tooth.

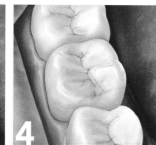

4 Note how beautifully the porcelain onlay blends in with the natural teeth.

3

CROWNS

The first molar shows extensive decay, requiring a full crown.

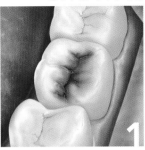

The decay is removed and part of the tooth rebuilt before final preparation and impression for the full crown.

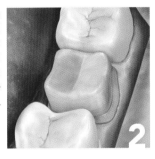

A porcelain crown is constructed in the lab and fit at the next visit.

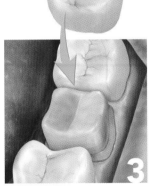

The final porcelain crown has been cemented in place.

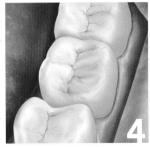

WHAT YOU SHOULD KNOW

MAKING RESTORATIONS LAST

Nothing lasts forever, including dental restorations. Dental materials are subject to not only chipping and fracturing but also everyday wear. Some people grind their teeth; others brush too vigorously. Even normal chewing eventually causes breakdown. The materials used to bond the restorations to the teeth can also deteriorate when exposed to oral fluids over long periods of time.

If you have dental restorations, avoid foods that may damage the bond of the restoration to the tooth, such as mints, chewing gum, candies, and other sticky, refined carbohydrates. Also make sure you don't clench or grind your teeth. Nothing causes more harm to new fillings or crowns. Although this tends to happen during sleep, it also can occur subconsciously during the day when you're concentrating or tense. Ask your dentist if you need a nightguard or any type of appliance to wear at night or during the day to protect your smile.

WHICH SOLUTION IS BEST FOR **YOU?**

COMPOSITE FILLING	INLAYS or ONLAYS
TREATMENT TIME	
Approximately 1 hour per tooth	Usually 2 office visits; 1–2 hours each per tooth
MAINTENANCE	
• Brush and floss daily.	• Brush and floss daily.
• Use a fluoride toothpaste and mouthwash as prescribed by your dentist.	• Use a fluoride toothpaste and mouthwash as prescribed by your dentist.
• Avoid biting down on hard foods and ice.	• Reduce intake of refined sugars and chewy foods such as caramels.
RESULTS	
• Esthetic replacement of old silver fillings or new decay areas	• More conservative than a full crown.
• May not be perfect color blend but much improved over metal surfaces	• Gold is most functional and longest-lasting method of restoring teeth, but large restorations tend to show metal.
	• Porcelain can be a highly esthetic replacement for discolored or metal posterior fillings.
	• Composite resin can match tooth color well.
TREATMENT LONGEVITY*	
5–8 years	*Gold:* 6–20 years
	Porcelain: 5–15 years
	Composite resin: 5–12 years
COST†	
$250 to $950 per tooth	*Gold:* $950 to $1,950 per tooth
	Porcelain: $850 to $2,200 per tooth
	Composite resin: $1,100 to $4,500 per tooth
ADVANTAGES	
• Esthetic (tooth-colored)	• Well-suited for large cavities
• Insulating	*Gold:*
• Completed in 1 office visit	• Longest lasting
• Extremely good bond to tooth structure	• Wears more like tooth structure
• Less expensive than crowns or inlays	• Will not fracture
• More conservative than crowns because less tooth reduction required	*Porcelain:*
	• Esthetic (tooth-colored)
	• Stronger than posterior composite resins
	• Extremely good bond to tooth structure
	• Will not stain
	• Insulating
	Composite resin:
	• May be less expensive than other options
DISADVANTAGES	
• More expensive than amalgam	• More expensive than amalgam
• Wears easily	*Gold:*
• Can stain, chip, or fracture	• Metal can show
• May have a shorter life expectancy than silver, gold, or porcelain	• Takes 2 office visits
• Less suited for large cavities	• Noninsulating (conducts heat and cold)
	Porcelain:
	• Can fracture
	• Takes 2 office visits (unless it is designed and created by machine in the dentist's office)
	• Possible wear of opposing natural tooth
	Composite resin:
	• Wears faster

*This estimate is based on the author's clinical experience combined with three university research studies and insurance company estimates. Your own experience could be different, depending on many factors, only some of which you and your dentist can control.

†Fees will vary from dentist to dentist based on the difficulty of the procedure, patient problems, patient dental and medical history, expectations, and dentist qualifications, including technical and artistic expertise.

‡Expect to pay extra for esthetic temporaries.

3

PORCELAIN VENEERS	CROWNS
2 office visits; 4 hours each	2–3 office visits; 1–2 hours each per tooth
• Avoid use of ultrasonic scaler and air abrasives during hygiene office visits. • Brush and floss daily. • Use a fluoride toothpaste and mouthwash as prescribed by your dentist. • Reduce intake of refined sugars and chewy foods such as caramels.	• Brush and floss daily. • Use a fluoride toothpaste and mouthwash as prescribed by your dentist. • Reduce intake of refined sugars and chewy foods such as caramels.
Can be highly esthetic but eventually may darken if the underlying tooth structure becomes darker.	Can achieve the best results in tooth shade, shape, and size.
5–12 years	5–15 years
$950 to $3,500 per tooth[‡]	$1,000 to $3,500 per tooth[‡]
• Excellent bond to enamel. • Less tooth reduction required than crowning. • Color change is possible. • Less staining than bonding.	• The dentist can improve shape of teeth. • Some realignment or straightening of teeth is possible. • Can be all-ceramic. • The greatest esthetic change is possible with this option.
• Difficult to repair if the veneer cracks or chips. • Irreversible if much enamel is removed. • Staining can occur between the porcelain and the margin of the tooth. • Cannot be lightened or bleached.	• Can fracture. • Requires an anesthetic. • Involves reduction of a significant amount of tooth structure. • More expensive than amalgam. • May decay if cement washes out.

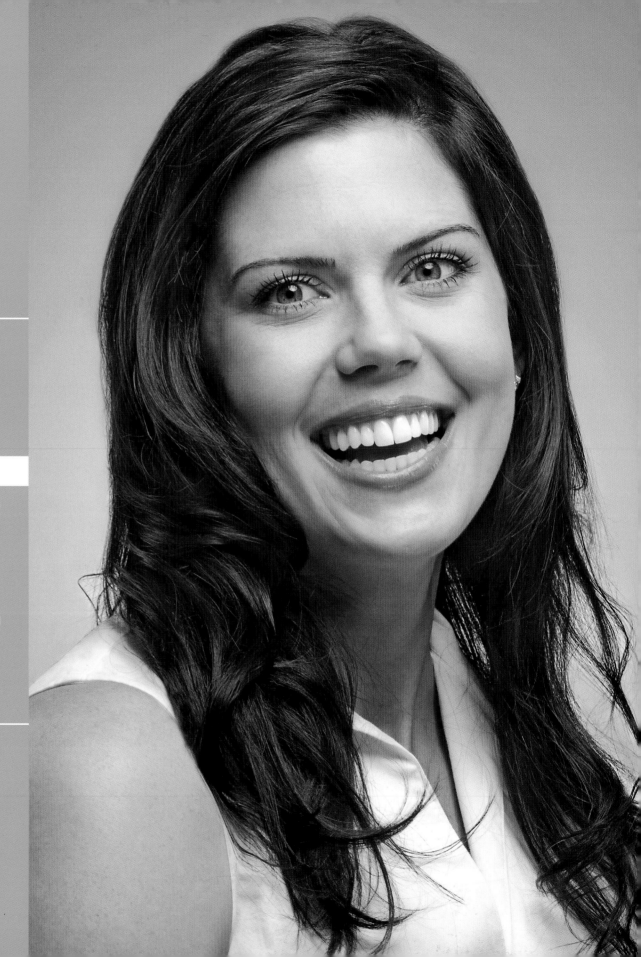

Cracking Down

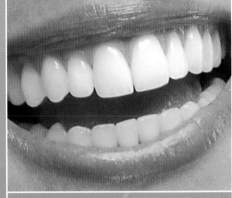

Why repair a broken tooth?

Many people who aren't aware of the consequences of not repairing chipped or broken teeth, or who are fearful of what restored teeth may look or feel like, choose to let their damaged teeth simply go unrepaired. The purpose of this chapter is to set the record straight.

A damaged tooth can be saved and repaired to look and feel like the real thing—perhaps even better! There are several treatment options available. The better informed you are about each of them, the more likely you are to be pleased with the results.

When a tooth gets chipped or fractured, the first consideration must be whether the pulp—the vital, living portion of the tooth—has been damaged. If a fracture is sensitive, painful, or uncomfortable, it may be because the pulp is exposed. Ultimately, the condition of the pulp and the amount of remaining tooth structure will determine the choice of treatment.

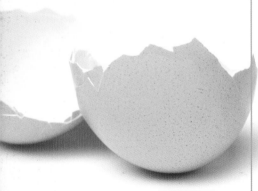

smile 101 What kind of fracture do you have?

Minor fracture

Minor fractures, such as small chips off the biting edges of the teeth, are usually simple to repair. If the chipped tooth is of sufficient length, it may be cosmetically contoured. Often, the neighboring teeth are also contoured so that no one tooth stands out from the rest. Or, an acid-etch bonding technique may be used to "fill out" the defect. Crowning should be avoided in cases of minor fracture whenever possible. Remember that it is always best—at least initially—to try simple therapies that preserve the color, shape, and health of the tooth.

Porcelain crown fracture

A porcelain crown fracture may also occur. Keep an eye on your metal-bonded crowns to see if dark outlines appear at the gum line. If a dark outline gradually appears, you may have a fracture of the crown or shrinkage of the gum tissue. If a fracture has occurred, the loss of porcelain at the gum line may weaken the remaining restoration, making it susceptible to additional damage. Eventually, the entire crown may have to be replaced. When detected early, however, some of these minor fractures can be repaired simply by smoothing the chipped porcelain or bonding composite resin to the area.

Serious fracture

Serious fractures, which are often caused by accidents, are best treated with the least amount of additional stress possible. Your dentist may choose to bond some teeth and crown others, especially when time is needed to determine if the nerves in the teeth can be saved. If you have a serious fracture, see your dentist as soon as possible, even if you aren't experiencing any pain. Often, the only sign of pulpal damage is tooth discoloration. In such cases, the damaged nerve is replaced with a root canal filling. Then, because much of the natural tooth structure is gone, full crowns typically are placed. If your tooth breaks at the gum line, your dentist may suggest cosmetic gum surgery to reveal more of your tooth root, which may allow your tooth to be saved and restored with a new crown.

Vertical root fracture

In cases of vertical root fracture, there may be no practical way to save the tooth, making extraction the only answer. However, all possibilities should be considered before any tooth is extracted. The goal is to maintain the integrity of the dental arch and to preserve the natural tooth as much as possible. In the event your tooth does need to be extracted, consider the possibility of an immediate implant replacement.

Immediate and beautiful results » This 45-year-old housewife fractured her right front central incisor and needed an immediate repair. The quickest and most esthetic repair is usually direct bonding of the fractured tooth. Note how natural and polished the final result is.

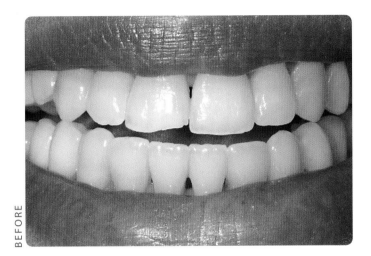

BEFORE

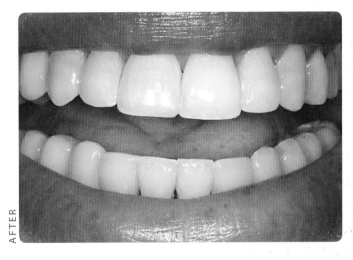

AFTER

expert tip An ounce of prevention . . .

Don't forget your mouth guard!

There's no way to anticipate most events that cause tooth fractures. Sports, however, are an exception. If you or someone you care about is involved in any type of contact sport, ask your dentist about a mouth guard. When designed and worn properly, mouth guards substantially reduce the risk of tooth fractures.

Watch out for microcracks!

Another good way to help prevent tooth fractures is to ask your dentist to perform an exam using an intraoral camera that reveals tiny microcracks. If these are associated with an old filling, it is usually best to replace the filling with one that incorporates the microcrack to help protect the tooth from further fracture. Until this has been done, be very careful to avoid biting down using the weakened tooth. Too often patients fracture teeth when biting down with a microcracked tooth on raspberries, blackberries, or other small-seeded or hard food items.

Solution 1 Cosmetic Contouring

WANT A SIMPLE SOLUTION?

Cosmetic contouring is an ideal treatment for small fractures and chips because an anesthetic is not required and the amount of tooth reduction involved is minimal—the rough edges are simply smoothed out. Once treatment is complete, few touch-ups are necessary. The cost and time involved are minimal as well.

is COSMETIC CONTOURING RIGHT FOR ME?

Cosmetic contouring is a cost-effective and minimally invasive way to repair small chips or fractures in teeth. Cosmetic contouring may be the best option if you:

- Have a very small fracture or chip in your tooth
- Want to invest a minimal amount of time and money in the procedure
- Have teeth that are long enough that contouring will not make them appear too short, aged, and/or worn

smile 101 Contouring provides a finishing touch

Although in some cases cosmetic contouring is an ideal treatment by itself, it also can be useful in conjunction with most other esthetic procedures. For example, if you are having one or more of your teeth treated with bonding, veneers, or crowns, your dentist can cosmetically contour adjacent or opposing teeth to create a more attractive and harmonious smile line. Also, cosmetic contouring often is used as a final touch following orthodontic treatment.

4

Fix it and forget it! » This 23-year-old woman chipped her front tooth on a metal object. She did not like the thought of losing more enamel or the constant maintenance that can be required with a bonded restoration. Since the two front teeth were more than adequate in length, it was determined that cosmetic contouring of both central incisors would be the ideal treatment.

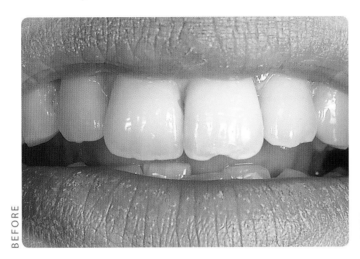

BEFORE

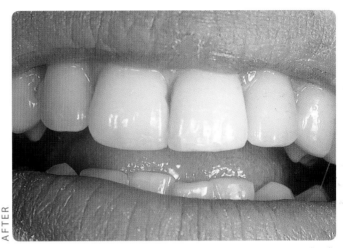

AFTER

WHAT YOU SHOULD KNOW

CONTOURING MAY AGE YOUR SMILE

Cosmetic contouring may not be the best treatment alternative for short teeth. If a chipped tooth is contoured, its neighbors are usually also contoured to match, which may flatten the entire smile line—the same thing that happens during the natural aging process as the teeth wear away. The result may be an older look. In such cases, bonding or laminating with porcelain would be a better alternative. Why add years to your smile unnecessarily?

Solution 2 Bonding

CAN BONDING IMPROVE YOUR SMILE?

There was a time when chipping a tooth meant replacing it with a crown, unless the chip was small enough to be cosmetically contoured. With bonding, however, a tooth can be restored simply by applying composite resin to its remaining structure. This rebuilds the tooth to its original shape, and often makes it look even better! The procedure also can be performed less expensively than placing veneers or crowns and typically in no more than an hour per tooth.

> How It's Done
> *see page 217*

is BONDING RIGHT FOR ME?

Bonding is by far the most desirable treatment when the tooth can be rebuilt without harming the smile line. Its primary drawback is that it may need to be repeated every 5 to 8 years because of stain and wear. If your tooth structure is still intact, improved bonding materials may provide you with stronger, longer-lasting, and more stain-resistant restorations in years to come. Once your tooth is reduced for a crown, you no longer have this alternative. Bonding may be the best option if you:

- Have a chip or fracture that is too large or teeth that are too short to allow cosmetic contouring
- Need emergency treatment for a complex fracture
- Want to avoid the expense and loss of tooth structure associated with crowns

Keep that youthful smile! » This 18-year-old model suffered a horizontal fracture of her right central incisor. In such cases, there are two choices: shorten the adjacent tooth through cosmetic contouring or bond the fractured tooth. Shortening the longer tooth would have meant changing the smile line and giving this model a less youthful look, so composite resin bonding was chosen to repair and lengthen the right front tooth.

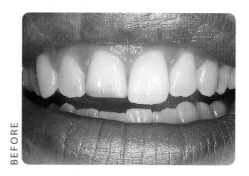

BEFORE

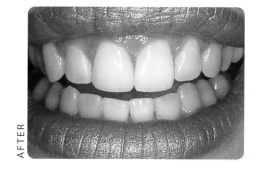

AFTER

4

Keep it simple! » This 17-year-old student and model fractured her two front teeth on the edge of a concrete swimming pool. Although the teeth were sensitive, the nerves remained intact. No anesthetic was required to slightly reshape the teeth and replace the missing parts with composite resin bonding material. Five years later, no additional treatment had been required for these teeth other than to replace the bonding once.

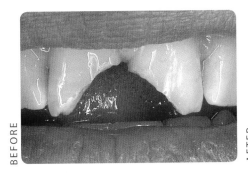

BEFORE

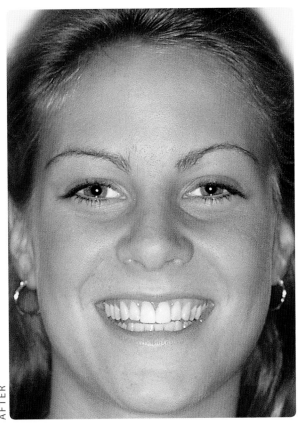

AFTER

BONDING MAY SAVE YOUR TEETH

Bonding can be used as a stop-gap measure in cases of complex fracture. By immediately sealing off exposed nerve endings with a sedative dressing and bonding material, your dentist may be able to preserve the nerve system in the tooth. This technique should be used in lieu of crowning whenever possible, particularly on front teeth.

smile 101 Bonding: A conservative option

The beauty of bonding is that little or no tooth structure needs to be removed to allow the composite resin to adhere to the dentin and enamel. For this reason, composite resin bonding is most often the technique of choice when esthetic dental restorative treatment is required.

Solution 3 Porcelain Veneers

WHAT ABOUT PORCELAIN VENEERS?

Although bonding is a quicker and more cost-effective treatment alternative than porcelain veneers, if your adjacent teeth have been rebuilt in porcelain, your fractured tooth should be restored in porcelain. The fractured tooth will match the adjacent teeth more closely because the same material has been used. Porcelain veneers or crowns may also be a preferred option if there are multiple teeth to be restored.

> ▶ How It's Done
> *see pages 218–219*

4

Beauty restored with multiple porcelain veneers » This 21-year-old student sustained multiple tooth fractures in an automobile accident. Emergency bonding with composite resin was maintained for a year to first determine which, if any, teeth would need root canal therapy. The lower teeth were bleached, then the bonding on the upper teeth was replaced by porcelain veneers, shown here. A bite guard should be worn at night to help protect the porcelain veneers from fracture due to possible clenching or grinding during sleep.

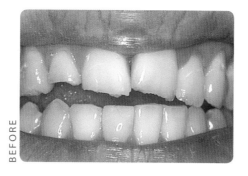

BEFORE

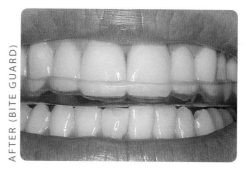

AFTER (BITE GUARD)

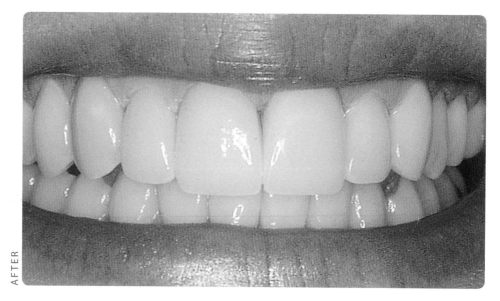

AFTER

are CROWNS RIGHT FOR ME?

Crowns offer an esthetic solution when little tooth structure remains following a fracture. Crowns may be the best option if you:

- Have lost too much tooth structure to allow contouring or bonding
- Are willing and able to spend more time and money on the procedure
- Want an esthetic solution that allows change in tooth shade and shape

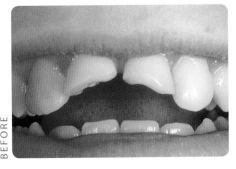

BEFORE

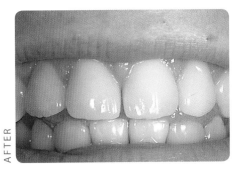

AFTER

A tooth is a terrible thing to waste! » This 12-year-old girl was referred to an oral surgeon to have her fractured teeth removed. Fortunately, the oral surgeon believed the teeth should be saved. Two metal posts were inserted, then the front teeth were crowned. Never assume that severely fractured teeth have to be extracted—it may be possible to save them.

WHEN IS A CROWN THE BEST OPTION?

If you fracture a front tooth so badly that there is little tooth structure left, a crown is probably the treatment of choice. If a back tooth fractures, it also may be best to restore it with a crown. The procedure should be performed immediately, especially if the pulp is exposed and living nerves are unprotected.

▶ How It's Done
see pages 220–225

Can crowns look natural? » This 19-year-old student fractured two of her teeth to such an extent that the nerves had to be removed. Posts were inserted, and two crowns were placed. Note how the form, texture, and highlights match the other teeth and create a natural appearance.

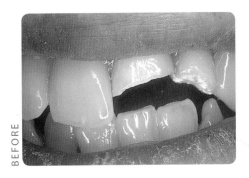

BEFORE

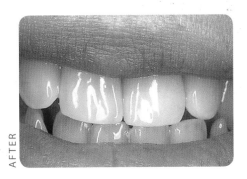

AFTER

WHICH SOLUTION IS BEST FOR **YOU?**

	COSMETIC CONTOURING	BONDING
TREATMENT TIME	15–60 min	1 hour per tooth
MAINTENANCE	Brush and floss daily.	• Have a professional cleaning 3–4 times per year. • Avoid biting down on hard foods and ice, and floss carefully as these teeth can chip easily. • See dentist for polishing or repair as necessary. • Get yearly fluoride treatments.
RESULTS	Teeth can appear straighter immediately after treatment.	Most fractures and chips are easliy repaired.
TREATMENT LONGEVITY*	Indefinite	5–8 years, with professional finishing once every few years
COST†	$200 to $2,500 per arch	$350 to $1,800 per tooth
ADVANTAGES	• No anesthetic required • Permanent results • No maintenance • Most conservative option • Quickest option	• No anesthetic required. • Little tooth reduction required. • Immediate results. • Teeth can be lightened. • Less expensive than veneers or crowns.
DISADVANTAGES	• Too much reduction can adversely affect the smile line. • Your bite may limit how much of the tooth can be removed. • In rare instances, sensitivity may be a problem.	• Can chip or stain • Has a limited esthetic life • May not be effective for severe fractures

*This estimate is based on the author's clinical experience combined with three university research studies and insurance company estimates. Your own experience could be different, depending on many factors, only some of which you and your dentist can control.

†Fees will vary from dentist to dentist based on the difficulty of the procedure, patient problems, patient dental and medical history, expectations, and dentist qualifications, including technical and artistic expertise.

‡Expect to pay extra for esthetic temporaries.

4

PORCELAIN VENEERS	CROWNS
2 office visits; 1 hour or more per tooth	Usually 2 office visits; 1–4 hours on up to 4 teeth (more time needed for additional teeth or more extensive treatment)
• Have a professional cleaning 2–4 times per year. • Avoid the use of ultrasonic scalers and air abrasives during hygiene office visits. • Take special care when biting into or chewing any hard foods. Use your back teeth to avoid placing torque on the veneer. • Get yearly fluoride treatments.	• Avoid biting down on hard foods and ice. • Get yearly fluoride treatments. • Brush and floss daily. • Brush your teeth properly to avoid gum recession that may expose the margin of your crown.
Fractured teeth can be restored or even improved.	Badly fractured teeth can be repaired and reshaped as desired.
5–12 years	5–15 years (directly related to fracture, problems with tissues, and decay)
$950 to $3,500 per tooth‡	Approximately $950 to $3,500 per tooth‡; expect to pay much more if a front tooth must be matched to other teeth
• Less chipping than bonding. • Color change is possible. • Excellent bond to enamel. • Gum tissue tolerates porcelain well. • Can improve entire smile if treating more teeth.	• The dentist can repair the chipped or fractured tooth. • Teeth can be lightened to any shade. • Some realignment or straightening of teeth is possible.
• More expensive than bonding. • Difficult to repair if the veneer cracks or chips. • Staining may occur between teeth, depending on how the veneer is prepared. • Irreversible if much enamel is removed. • Usually requires an anesthetic .	• Can fracture. • Requires an anesthetic. • Tooth form is altered (most of the tooth enamel is removed). • Not a permanent solution. • More expensive than bonding.

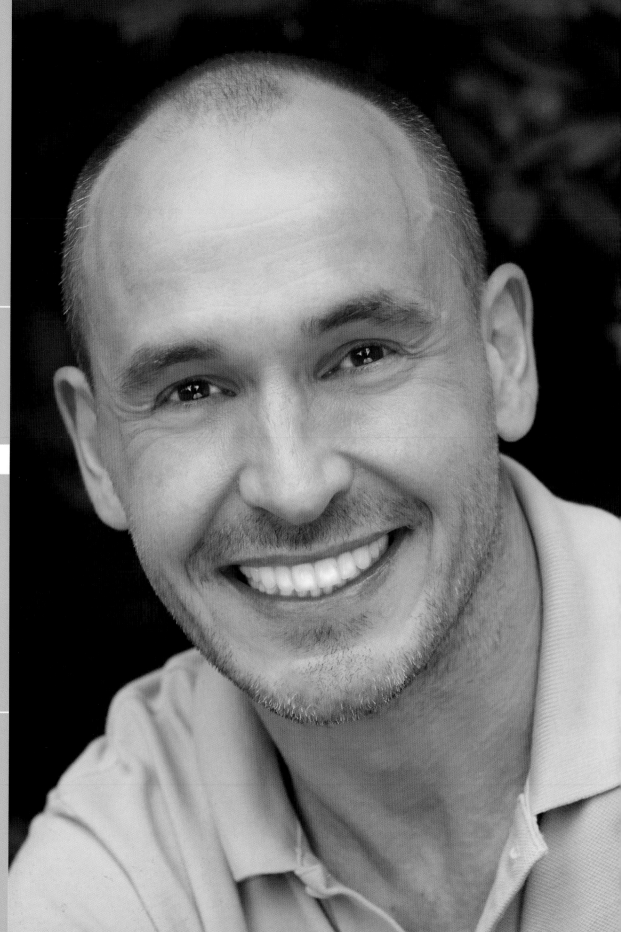

5

Mind the Gap

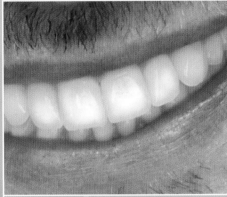

Eliminate spaces between your teeth for the ultimate makeover.

Many people don't realize the effect a space between the front teeth can have on a person's appearance. Consider the story of a man in his 40s who had a gap closed between his upper front teeth. A week after the crowns were placed he said, "Some of my friends thought I had a new hairstyle. Others actually thought I'd had a face-lift! They don't realize that the only thing different is that the space between my front teeth is gone." This same phenomenon happens over and over again. Why? Because for the first time, people are actually looking at the person's face instead of the space between his or her teeth.

If you have a space between your teeth that you don't like, but you haven't had it closed because you were told it would take years of orthodontic treatment, this chapter is for you. In addition to orthodontics, spaces between teeth can be corrected with bonding, porcelain veneers, or all-ceramic crowns. But don't be surprised if people don't recognize exactly what's different about you. Just get ready for comments like, "You look terrific!"

WHAT
CAUSES GAPS?

Spaces between the teeth are most often caused by heredity. However, they also may be caused by personal habits such as tongue thrusting or by abnormal tongue or swallowing movements. The loss of bone under the gum tissue can also cause teeth to separate, as can loss of the back teeth, which often transfers chewing activity forward. How a space is treated has a lot to do with its cause.

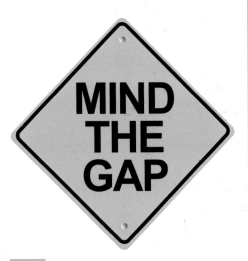

smile 101 Remember the three *R*s!

There are several ways to close unsightly gaps. Which method is chosen depends on the cause of the space, its size, its location, and the condition of adjacent teeth. Both cost and your personal needs will play a significant role in your choice of treatment. Correcting space problems, however, usually involves one of the three *R*s:

- Repositioning teeth with orthodontics. When teeth are attractive and healthy, repositioning is the ideal treatment, as it involves no loss of enamel. Some alternatives, such as full crowns, require sacrificing healthy tooth structure for cosmetic correction.

- Restoring teeth through bonding, veneers, or crowns. Patients frequently prefer immediate results. In such cases, bonding or laminating with porcelain may be the answer. In other cases, a combination of therapies offers the best results.

- Removal of teeth, followed by replacement with a bridge or implant. Removal is used only as a last resort and will not be covered in this chapter. See the next chapter for more information on replacing missing teeth.

After you read this chapter, you will be in a much better position to talk with your dentist about which option is best for you. Just keep in mind that the goal of treatment is always to fill the space while avoiding the loss of teeth or tooth structure as much as possible.

expert tip First things first!

If the gaps in your smile are caused by gum disease, it's important to resolve this underlying problem before beginning any other treatment.

Looking for a temporary fix for your smile?

The removable acrylic overlay is a device formed from thin acrylic or plastic made to cover the space and blend with adjacent teeth. It's easily snapped in, and the intimate fit of the appliance to the teeth holds it in place. Removable acrylic overlays were more commonly used before the advent of bonding. They were often worn by models, actors, and others who didn't want to crown their teeth just to close a space.

While these overlays may look attractive from a distance, they often don't bear up well under close scrutiny. They add bulk to the natural teeth, so are kept as thin as possible. However, because the plastic is so thin, it's difficult to make overlays look natural, and they can fracture and discolor easily. Moreover, eating with them can be a problem.

In some cases, however, the removable acrylic overlay may still be a desirable alternative. On the positive side, it's inexpensive, and it hides spaces well, particularly for photographic purposes. If you have a special event coming up or just want a trial smile to see how you would look without your gap, talk to your dentist about getting a removable acrylic overlay.

A smile for special occasions » This 52-year-old woman wanted to have her spaces closed for certain occasions, such as when being photographed, but she did not want to have her teeth altered with restorations or orthodontic treatment, nor did she want to close the space permanently.

A removable acrylic overlay was made to snap into place, giving the patient immediate results without permanently altering her tooth structure. This allows the option of orthodontics or any other type of treatment later. The disadvantage of this type of removable appliance is that the plastic teeth are extremely thin, fragile, and easily fractured.

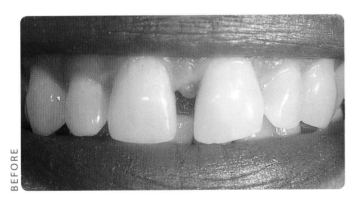

BEFORE

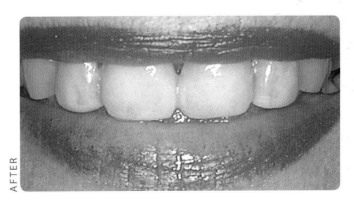

AFTER

Solution 1 Orthodontics

ADULTS DO WEAR BRACES!

Braces aren't just for kids anymore. In fact, adults now comprise more than 20% of patients who seek the help of an orthodontist. In some cases, treatment consists of only removable appliances or retainers. In others, clear or tooth-colored brackets, instead of traditional metal ones, can be used, or a patient may choose a system using clear matrices (such as Invisalign) or lingual braces, which are mounted behind the teeth.

▶ How It's Done
see page 231

is ORTHODONTICS RIGHT FOR ME?

Orthodontics is a long-lasting, conservative approach to closing unsightly spaces between teeth. New techniques that are almost invisible have removed some of the stigma of having braces; however, orthodontics does take longer than most of the other options. Orthodontics may be the best option if you:

- Want to use the most conservative method, in terms of cost and loss of tooth structure
- Are willing to invest time in the procedure
- Don't mind some compromise of esthetics during treatment
- Will agree to wear your retainer at night indefinitely
- Have otherwise healthy and attractive teeth

expert tip   You don't have to wait!

As a compromise, you may consider moving the teeth to a more favorable (if not ideal) position in just a few months, then bonding or placing veneers on them in this improved position. The advantage to this is being able to give the teeth better proportions.

5

WHAT YOU SHOULD KNOW

ORTHODONTICS IS USUALLY BEST

In the long run, orthodontics is the best solution for most people. Even if full crowns eventually will be needed, teeth should be aligned properly first. And although orthodontic treatment requires regular adjustments and the most time of the alternatives—usually taking 6 months to 2 years to complete—it has the advantage of leaving the natural teeth intact and being close to a permanent solution (although in most cases, retainers must be worn to keep teeth from shifting back to their original positions). Bonding, porcelain veneers, or crowns, on the other hand, will usually require repair or periodic replacement.

Not your kid's braces » This network television correspondent had a large gap between his front teeth. Because television tends to magnify the size of a space, it was desirable to have the space closed. The teeth also were off center, causing a midline deviation. Tooth-colored wire and plastic brackets were used because of the esthetic demands of this patient's vocation. Viewers did not even realize he was undergoing orthodontic treatment because of the near invisibility of these appliances from a distance. About 18 months were required to produce this more flattering smile using orthodontics. The final step was to bond the front teeth together with composite resin to keep the space from returning. Notice how no attention is called to the now seemingly minor midline deviation. Orthodontic movement improved his smile as well as his bite.

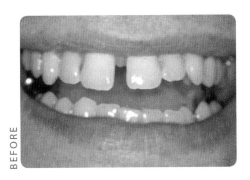

BEFORE

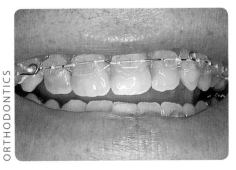

ORTHODONTICS

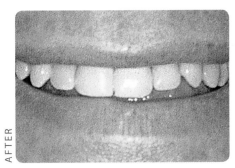

AFTER

Solution 2 Bonding

HOW DOES BONDING WORK?

Composite resin, a plastic material, is applied to etched enamel to make the teeth wider in areas where gaps exist. Bonding may also be used to close a space temporarily, for example, until crowns are made or during orthodontic treatment. The procedure can be performed without an anesthetic in one office visit.

> How It's Done
> *see page 217*

Simple solutions can have great effects » This 29-year-old sales executive had lost a lower tooth, causing the teeth to shift and creating unattractive spaces that showed when he talked or smiled. The upper incisors were also uneven and chipped.

In one appointment, composite resin bonding and cosmetic contouring of the upper and lower incisors greatly improved his smile. Even though there are only three lower incisors, they look good because they are in proper balance with the rest of the mouth. A new smile helped this man improve his life through a better job. Research has shown that when people feel confident, their outlook on life and their ability to achieve are enhanced.

BEFORE
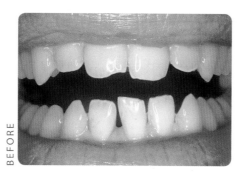

AFTER
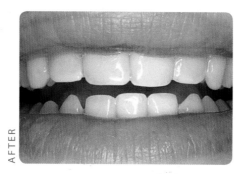

AFTER
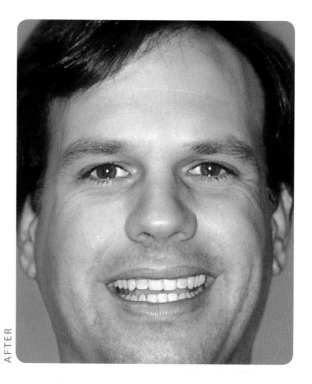

5

is BONDING RIGHT FOR ME?

In recent years, bonding has proved to be a highly effective treatment for closing spaces between the teeth. Bonding may be the best option if you:

- Want immediate results
- Desire a less expensive and less invasive option than veneers or crowns
- Have other esthetic problems that could be solved by bonding
- Prefer a procedure that is reversible

expert tip Don't stop with the gap!

If you are closing gaps with bonding, also consider taking care of any other visible defects such as rotated or broken teeth at the same time. If some of your teeth are too dark, bonding can be used to lighten them while also closing any gaps.

Bonding for a whole new smile »
This newspaper columnist and author had large spaces between her front teeth to the extent that her teeth were "flaring out." This caused a reverse smile line—the edges of her canines were lower than the edges of her central incisors. The teeth were different colors; many of them were too yellow and stained. Finally, the protruding upper right canine overlapped the tooth behind it.

All of the front teeth were bonded with composite resin to lighten the teeth as well as close the spaces between them. The teeth were also lengthened to help achieve a younger-looking smile line. Cosmetic contouring helped to create a more harmonious relationship between the teeth. The entire treatment was done in one appointment.

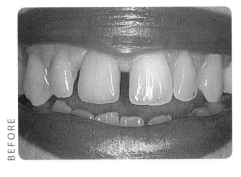

BEFORE

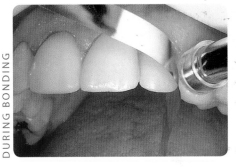

DURING BONDING

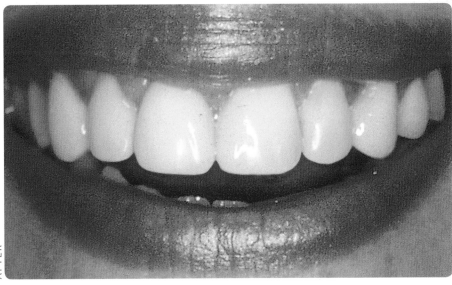

AFTER

75

A sneak peek at your new smile » This attractive 28-year-old dentist disliked smiling because of the spaces between her teeth. A wax-up revealed how her smile would look with bonded resin to close the spaces. An entirely new look for her smile was accomplished with direct composite resin bonding in just one appointment. Now this dentist uses her smile to inspire others to achieve the smile of their dreams.

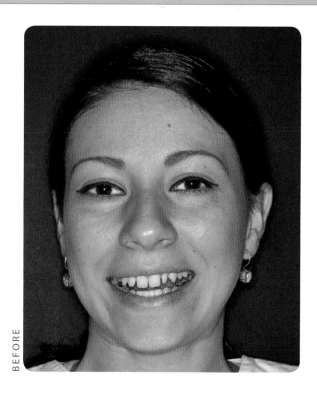

BEFORE

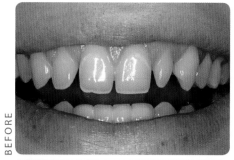

BEFORE

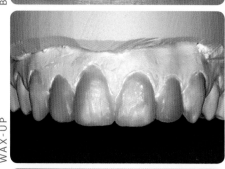

WAX-UP

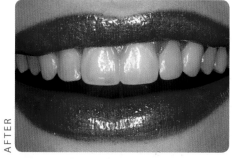

AFTER

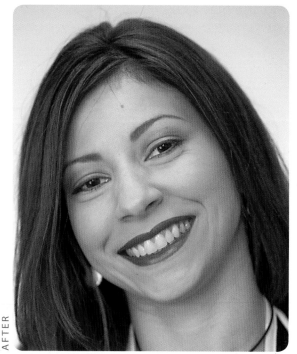

AFTER

5

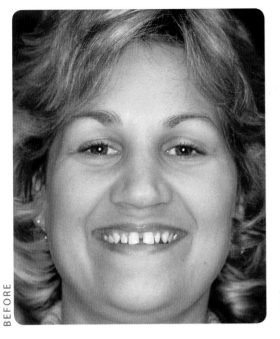

BEFORE

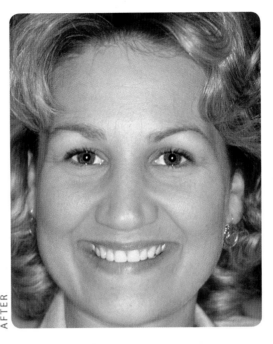

AFTER

Small teeth can cause big gaps » Although orthodontic treatment could have been used to close the spaces for this patient, the result would not have been ideal since her teeth were too small for her face. In one appointment, bonding closed the spaces and made the teeth more proportionate, giving her a more attractive smile. Bonding may be the ideal solution when gaps are caused by small teeth. However, treatment may require bonding more teeth than the ones actually affected to keep them in proportion. Otherwise, teeth may appear too bulky. This effect can be minimized if teeth are lengthened slightly and the edges are not perfectly even.

BOND ONLY HEALTHY TEETH

Gum disease or bone loss must be treated before bonding takes place. The only exception to this rule is when your dentist believes that the loose teeth need to be splinted together.

smile 101 Can I preview my new smile?

Computer imaging can help show you how many teeth will need treatment and the approximate results. If computer imaging does not provide enough information for you, ask your dentist to add tooth-colored wax to a model of your teeth so that you can get a better idea of the end result. Although there is a distinct difference between waxing and bonding because of the way light is reflected, this "mock-up" will give you some idea of how the final result will look. You can also ask your dentist to apply temporary bonding material directly on your teeth to get a good idea of how your smile will change.

BONDED TEETH
REQUIRE CARE

Bonding can be used successfully on both upper and lower teeth. However, bonded teeth are more likely to chip, crack, and stain than are natural teeth, particularly the lower front teeth, which are more susceptible to forces from chewing. This also means that some repairs to the bonding are considered normal maintenance during its life expectancy. If you have bonded teeth, a professional cleaning three to four times a year is a must. Even then, the bonding may need to be replaced or repaired in 5 to 8 years.

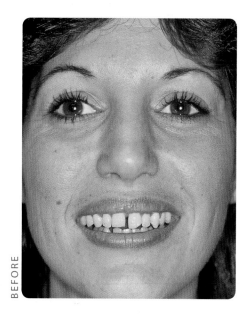

BEFORE

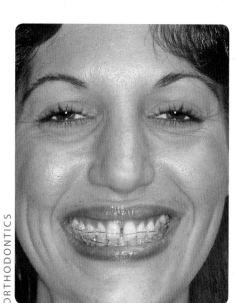

ORTHODONTICS

Combining treatments for an ideal result » This 33-year-old cosmetologist was concerned about her protruding teeth and the space between her front teeth. Orthodontic treatment using plastic brackets successfully retracted the teeth and closed the space. Although orthodontic treatment alone made her smile more attractive, a combination of cosmetic contouring and composite resin bonding further enhanced it. Looking your best can sometimes call for a combination of several treatments.

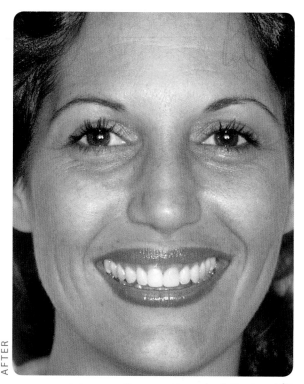

AFTER

Solution 3 Porcelain Veneers

are PORCELAIN VENEERS RIGHT FOR ME?

Porcelain veneers provide a more esthetic option compared with bonding. Porcelain veneers may be the best option if you:

- Consider esthetics to be more important than expense
- Are comfortable with the required enamel reduction
- Want to avoid the chipping that can occur with bonding as well as the higher expense of crowns

It's more than just a new smile » This 22-year-old waitress was too embarrassed to smile, which limited her full potential both socially and in reaching her career goals. Porcelain veneers and a resin-bonded fixed bridge were made without reducing the tooth structure. (This can best be accomplished when the teeth need building out or when multiple spaces exist.) The result was a life-changing physical transformation for this young woman, who is now a graduate student and one step closer to her goal of a business career.

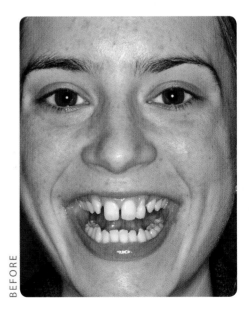

BEFORE

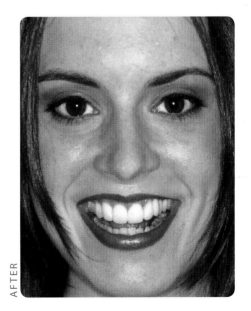

AFTER

WHY SPEND MORE FOR PORCELAIN VENEERS?

Although bonding is the quickest way to close spaces between the teeth, laminating with porcelain is also an option. Although veneers take at least two appointments and typically cost much more than bonding, a major advantage is the proportional accuracy that they provide. This technique is especially effective when spaces are not uniform. Another reason to choose porcelain veneers is that they will not stain nearly as much as bonded restorations.

> How It's Done
> *see pages 218–219*

Solution 4 Crowns

WHEN ARE CROWNS THE ANSWER?

Although crowns can provide beautiful results—filling gaps and lightening tooth color just like bonding—they typically are not the treatment of choice for spaces between the teeth because their placement requires considerable reduction of natural tooth structure. However, in cases where teeth are badly damaged, these finely sculptured look-alikes are often ideal.

> **How It's Done**
> *see pages 220–225*

are CROWNS RIGHT FOR ME?

In most cases, gaps between teeth are better addressed using less invasive procedures such as orthodontics or bonding. However, there are some circumstances in which crowns offer the best solution. Crowns may be the best option if you:

- Have teeth that are badly damaged
- Require or desire major changes in the shape or alignment of your teeth
- Feel comfortable with the higher cost and loss of tooth structure associated with crowns

what to eXpect CROWNS

Crowns are a more time-consuming and costly option than bonding or veneers. Crowns are not as likely to chip as veneers and bonding; however, replacement still may be required within 5 to 15 years.

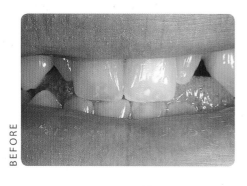
BEFORE

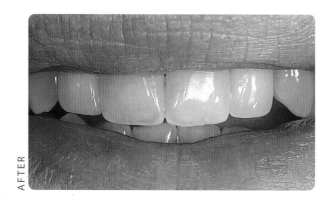
AFTER

Tooth size does matter! » This 35-year-old salesman had peg-shaped lateral incisors that created large gaps in his smile. He was so ashamed of his appearance he avoided smiling. The lateral incisors were crowned to improve the smile line. In similar situations, porcelain veneers or composite resin bonding often can be used as a more conservative means of altering tooth shape.

5

WHAT YOU SHOULD KNOW

IS A SMALL SPACE BETTER THAN LARGE CROWNS?

Occasionally, a space is so large that a patient prefers that a slight gap be left between the crowns. If the crowns were made large enough to completely fill the gap, they would appear unnatural and out of proportion with the other teeth. It is better to close the gap somewhat with orthodontics before placing the crowns. Another option is to consider including more teeth in the restoration plan to better apportion the space.

Oversized crowns: More harm than good » When this young lady smiled, she revealed two oversized crowns that had been placed to mask a sizeable gap between her two front teeth. These oversized crowns were reduced and left in place during orthodontic treatment to close the newly formed spaces. Two new porcelain crowns were made following orthodontic treatment to enhance her smile.

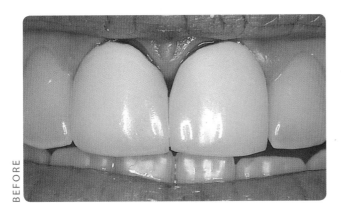

BEFORE

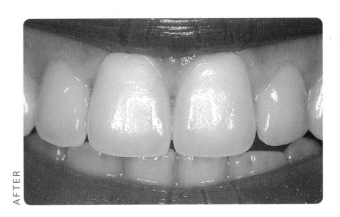

AFTER

WHICH SOLUTION IS BEST FOR **YOU?**

	ORTHODONTICS	BONDING
TREATMENT TIME	6–24 mo for most patients	1 office visit; 1–2 hours per tooth
MAINTENANCE	• Brush and floss daily. • Have a professional cleaning 3–4 times per year. • Wear retainers at night indefinitely, at least a few nights per week. • Use a water-powered device daily for thorough cleaning.	• Have a professional cleaning 3–4 times per year. • Avoid biting down with front teeth, especially on hard foods. • Brush and floss daily. • See dentist for polishing or repair as necessary.
RESULTS	Spaces between teeth are closed.	Most spaces can be filled in to look natural.
TREATMENT LONGEVITY*	Generally permanent if retainer is worn at least a few nights per week	5–8 years, with professional refinishing once every few years
COST†	$1,550 to $7,500, depending on the number of teeth involved and the appliance used	$350 to $1,800 per tooth
ADVANTAGES	• Closes space between teeth • Permanent results for most people if retainers are worn • No tooth reduction required • May be the least expensive option	• Little or no tooth reduction required. • No anesthetic required. • Reversible procedure. • Less expensive than veneers or crowns. • Color change is possible.
DISADVANTAGES	• Time-consuming. • Teeth may return to original position if retainers are not worn. • Thorough cleanings are more difficult during treatment.	• Can chip or stain more easily than veneers or crowns. • Has a limited esthetic life. • Treatment may involve extra teeth to obtain proportionate space closing. • Teeth may appear and feel thicker.

*This estimate is based on the author's clinical experience combined with three university research studies and insurance company estimates. Your own experience could be different, depending on many factors, only some of which you and your dentist can control.

†Fees will vary from dentist to dentist based on the difficulty of the procedure, patient problems, patient dental and medical history, expectations, and dentist qualifications, including technical and artistic expertise.

‡Expect to pay extra for esthetic temporaries.

5

PORCELAIN VENEERS	CROWNS
2 office visits; 1–4 hours each (more time needed for office visits, more extensive treatment)	2 office visits; 1–4 hours each for up to 4 teeth (more time needed for more extensive treatment)
• Have a professional cleaning 3–4 times per year. • Take special care when biting into or chewing hard foods. Use your back teeth to avoid placing torque on the veneer.	• Avoid biting down on hard foods and ice. • Get yearly fluoride treatments. • Brush and floss daily.
A polished, natural-appearing result that effectively closes spaces	The best method to improve tooth shapes to fill spaces
5–12 years if special care is taken	5–15 years (directly related to fractures, problems with tissues, and decay)
$950 to $3,500 per tooth‡	$950 to $3,500 per tooth‡
• Easier to obtain proportionate closure of spaces. • Less chipping and staining than bonding. • Less loss of color or luster. • Less tooth reduction required than crowning. • Lasts longer than bonding. • Gum tissue tolerates porcelain well. • Color change is possible.	• Can be shaped to esthetically fill gaps. • Teeth can be lightened to any shade. • Some realignment or straightening of teeth is possible. • Should last about twice as long as bonding. • Gum tissue tolerates porcelain well. • Color change is possible.
• More expensive than bonding • Difficult to repair if the veneer cracks or chips • Irreversible if much enamel is removed • May not be best choice in difficult bite situations	• Can fracture. • Requires an anesthetic. • Tooth form is altered (most of the tooth enamel is removed). • May need to be replaced after 5–15 years. • More expensive than bonding.

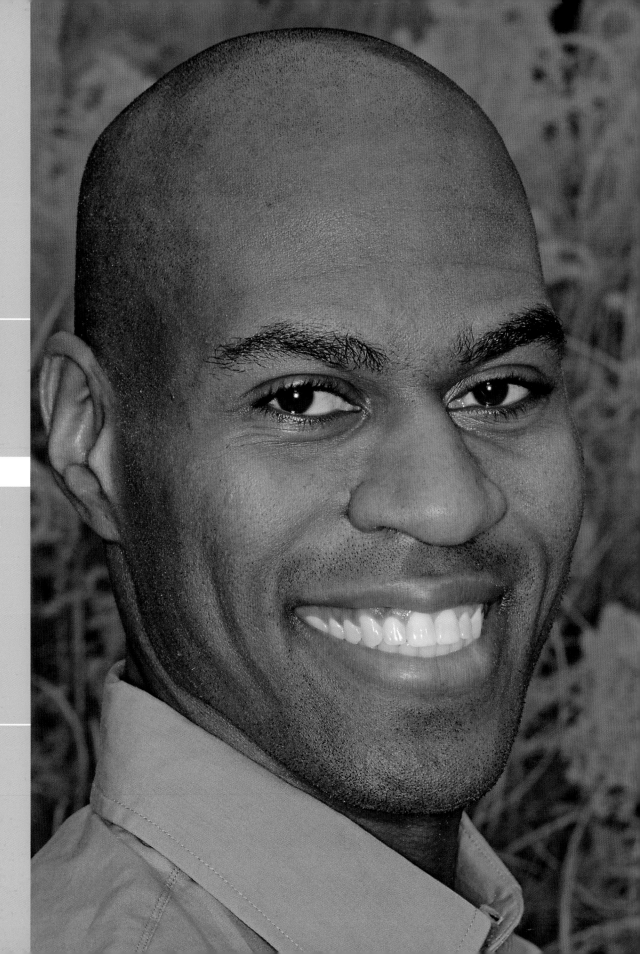

6

FIND OUT . . .

WHY IT'S IMPORTANT TO
REPLACE MISSING TEETH

HOW TO REGAIN YOUR
YOUTHFUL SMILE

IF IMPLANTS ARE
RIGHT FOR YOU

Lost and Found

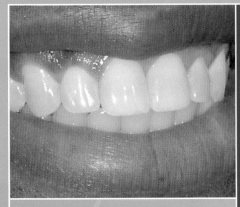

A missing tooth can spoil a good smile.

Don't underestimate the value of every tooth in terms of beauty—even those in the back of the mouth. Although the spaces created by missing teeth may not be visible, they can cause a variety of problems. For example, chewing forces may shift, causing the front teeth to flare out and create unwanted spaces. An altered bite can also cause the collapse of facial features. The more teeth that are lost and not replaced, the greater the odds that wrinkles and lines will form, causing premature aging. Only if the missing tooth is the last molar should it go unreplaced.

If you're missing one or more teeth, you have four options for making your smile complete: a fixed bridge, a removable bridge, a complete denture, or implants. Each can be successful, depending on your circumstances.

Solution 1 **Fixed Bridge**

WHAT IS A FIXED BRIDGE?

Fixed bridges (also called *fixed partial dentures*) are used to replace missing teeth and gum tissue. They are attached to neighboring teeth and cemented into place. The underlying substructure can be made of a ceramic material or metal, but the restorations are typically porcelain.

> How It's Done
see pages 226–227

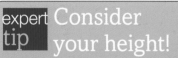
expert tip **Consider your height!**

If you are taller or shorter than average, an all-ceramic bridge may be the best choice. If others normally see you from either above or below, the metal on a bridge or crown is more likely to be visible.

6

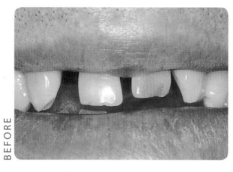
BEFORE

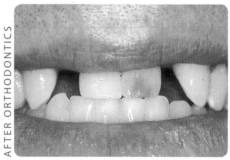
AFTER ORTHODONTICS

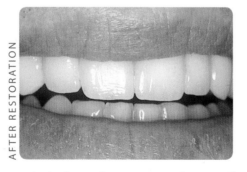
AFTER RESTORATION

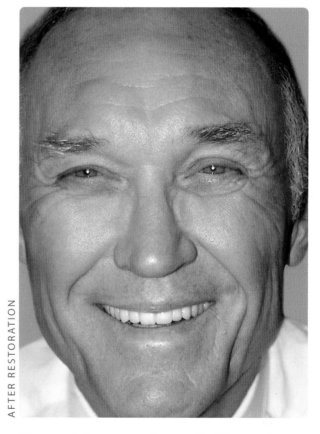
AFTER RESTORATION

It may take more than a bridge » This 50-year-old man wanted to enhance his appearance, but missing lateral incisors and irregular spacing created a problem too difficult to solve strictly through restorative therapy. The patient underwent 16 months of orthodontic treatment with tooth-colored brackets. Adequate space allowed proportionate restoration of his upper front teeth. The final restorative treatment consisted of fixed bridges and porcelain veneers on the upper teeth and in-office bleaching for the lower teeth. In this patient, combination therapy contributed to a proportionate, esthetic, and functional result.

is A FIXED BRIDGE RIGHT FOR ME?

Generally speaking, if you're missing a tooth or teeth, and if you have sufficient bone, dental implants are most often the best choice. However, a fixed bridge may be the best option if you:

- Have economic or health reasons that prevent you from getting implants
- Want an option that usually lasts longer and looks and feels better than a removable appliance
- Don't mind having adjacent teeth crowned to serve as an anchor

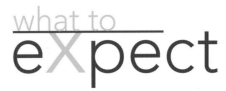

what to eXpect

BRIDGES WILL CHANGE THE WAY YOU FLOSS

It's important to remember that the teeth being replaced and used to support the bridge will be joined. This means you will no longer be able to floss through the contacts between the teeth. Instead, you will need a floss threader, which will allow you to floss under the missing tooth or teeth as well as between the teeth.

---

smile 101 How natural can a bridge look?

The greatest esthetic challenge dentists face when making bridges is giving the artificial teeth a natural look. It's difficult to make them look like individual teeth that are actually emerging from your gums. No matter how skilled dentists and laboratory technicians are, they will occasionally have difficulty in solving these problems.

WHAT YOU SHOULD KNOW

METAL VS CERAMIC FRAMEWORK

Porcelain can be bonded to a precious or nonprecious metal. Although precious metals such as gold are generally more expensive, some nonprecious metals can tarnish, leaving a slightly dark line near the gum tissue if the porcelain does not fully encase the metal. Zirconia or other very hard tooth-colored ceramic may be used instead to provide more translucency and naturalness. These new all-ceramic bridges offer more strength and improved esthetics.

WHAT YOU SHOULD KNOW

CONVENTIONAL FIXED BRIDGE

ADVANTAGES

- ▶ Long lasting
- ▶ Easy to clean
- ▶ Can improve your bite
- ▶ Helps prevent movement of adjacent and opposing teeth

DISADVANTAGES

- ▶ Costs more than removable bridge
- ▶ More tooth reduction than cantilever or resin-bonded bridge
- ▶ May be more difficult to achieve natural look in cases of bone or gum loss

what to eXpect

CONVENTIONAL FIXED BRIDGE

A beautiful esthetic result can be achieved with a conventional fixed bridge because the teeth needed to anchor the bridge on either side of the missing teeth are made into crowns and no metal shows. However, there must be sufficient room for porcelain between the upper and lower teeth when replacing a missing tooth with a fixed bridge. If necessary, either a crown-lengthening surgical procedure or orthodontic treatment can usually help create the needed space.

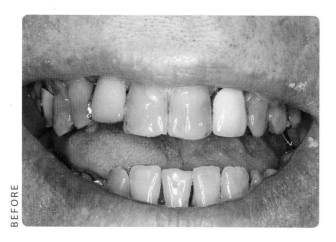

BEFORE

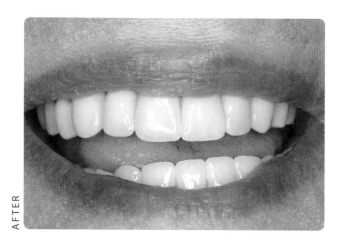

AFTER

No time for the dentist » This extremely successful businessman never seemed to have time to take care of his teeth. It took continuous effort by his devoted wife to convince him to have his smile treated. Placement of conventional fixed bridges and full crowns changed his smile forever. It is not uncommon for spouses to be the motivating factor behind a life-changing improvement in a smile.

6

What is a cantilever fixed bridge?

A cantilever fixed bridge is attached on only one side and therefore is an option when there is not an anchor tooth available on both sides of a tooth to be replaced. The cantilever fixed bridge may be considered a more conservative treatment than a conventional bridge because fewer teeth are reduced, and the esthetic result can be as good or better. It is also less expensive than a conventional bridge; however, its life expectancy is usually not as long.

WHAT YOU SHOULD KNOW

CANTILEVER FIXED BRIDGE

ADVANTAGES

► Less tooth structure reduced

► Less expensive than conventional bridge

► More natural separation possible between teeth

DISADVANTAGES

► Less structural support

► Unless the bite is perfectly balanced, too much torque can damage the replacement tooth

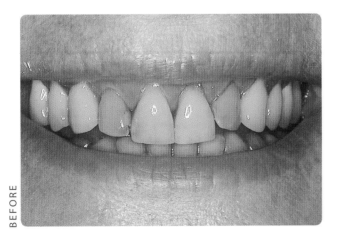

BEFORE

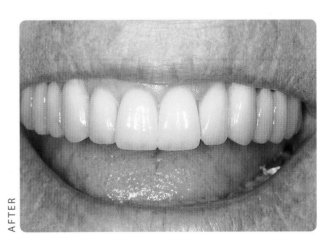

AFTER

Restoring form with function » This patient's upper molars had been extracted as a result of periodontal disease. In addition, she was not happy with her discolored front teeth. A 12-unit fixed cantilever bridge was constructed, not only replacing her missing first molars, but also giving her the smile she had long wanted.

WHAT YOU SHOULD KNOW

RESIN-BONDED FIXED BRIDGE

ADVANTAGES

▶ Less expensive than conventional bridge

▶ No anesthetic required

▶ Can improve your bite

▶ Little or no tooth reduction

DISADVANTAGES

▶ Less ability to alter shape and size of teeth

▶ Gum tissue can shrink around the replacement tooth, leaving spaces between teeth

▶ Metal backing may show through if the teeth are thin

▶ Teeth to which the bridge is attached must be in excellent condition

▶ Can become de-bonded much more easily than a fixed conventional bridge

▶ May not last as long as a conventional bridge

smile 101 What is a resin-bonded fixed bridge?

Another type of fixed bridge is the resin-bonded bridge, also called a *Maryland bridge*. The replacement tooth or teeth are attached to a metal framework that is bonded to adjacent teeth with resin cement. If the teeth adjacent to the missing tooth are intact and in good condition, this type of restoration may be a good choice. If there are cosmetic problems with the adjacent teeth, however, a conventional bridge should be considered.

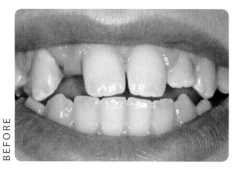
BEFORE

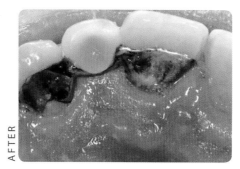
AFTER

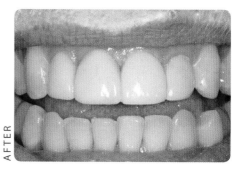
AFTER

Not quite ready for an implant? » Although this teenager ultimately wanted a dental implant to replace his missing tooth, the decision was made to delay implant placement until he was older, and a resin-bonded bridge was placed in the meantime. The bridge is attached to the inside of the adjacent teeth; therefore, little or no tooth structure is lost in the process. A correctly planned and placed resin-bonded bridge is an esthetic and conservative treatment option for missing teeth.

6

Solution 2 Removable Bridge

WHAT IS A REMOVABLE BRIDGE?

expert tip Take the long view!

Although patients often select the removable bridge over the fixed bridge because it's less expensive initially, this may not be a wise decision since removable bridges have shorter life spans. In addition, removable bridges often cause unnecessary wear and tear to adjacent teeth.

smile 101 You never have to be without your teeth!

Your dentist can make a natural-looking temporary bridge—even on the day you lose a tooth! However, the temporary bridge has a relatively short life expectancy and should be replaced with a final bridge as soon as healing takes place.

Like fixed bridges, removable bridges (also called *removable partial dentures*) replace missing teeth and gum tissue and are attached to neighboring teeth. However, they're not cemented into place and therefore can be removed. There are two basic types of removable bridges: conventional and precision attachment. Each is discussed in this section.

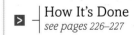
How It's Done
see pages 226–227

what to eXpect

REMOVABLE BRIDGE CONSTRUCTION

The framework for most removable bridges is made of a silver-colored nonprecious metal that has high strength and is tarnish resistant. Acrylic or porcelain teeth are then attached to this framework with gum-colored plastic so that the removable bridge looks as natural as possible.

WHAT YOU SHOULD KNOW

CONVENTIONAL REMOVABLE BRIDGE

ADVANTAGES

▶ Relatively inexpensive way to replace missing teeth

▶ Helps to balance bite and increases chewing efficiency by replacing missing teeth

▶ Prevents movements of adjacent and opposing teeth

DISADVANTAGES

▶ Clasps may cause wear and stress on supporting teeth

▶ Not the most esthetic option, especially when metal clasps are used

what to eXpect

CONVENTIONAL REMOVABLE BRIDGE

The conventional removable bridge attaches to adjacent teeth with metal clasps. If these clasps show when you smile, the result can be esthetically displeasing. In such cases, the precision-attachment removable bridge described next should be considered. If you can't afford the precision-attachment method of hiding clasps, then a removable bridge with a tooth-colored flexible clasp can be made to replace the missing teeth. Keep in mind, however, that this clasp doesn't offer the support or the stability of the conventional metal clasp, and the bridge may need to be replaced every few years.

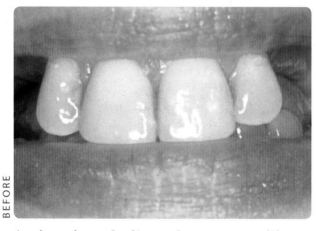

BEFORE

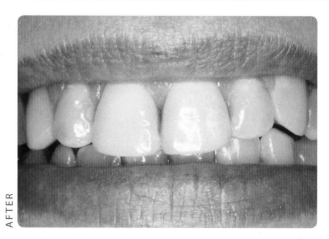

AFTER

An interim solution to keep you smiling » This woman had lost many of her upper back teeth. She avoided smiling in order to hide the spaces left by her missing teeth. At the time, she couldn't afford a fixed bridge and didn't want the metal clasps of a removable bridge to show in her smile. A removable bridge with tooth-colored clasps provided an esthetic interim solution for this patient. For the most esthetic and long-lasting result, implants or fixed bridges eventually should be placed.

6

smile 101 What is a precision attachment?

If you object to the metal clasps found in the conventional removable bridge, you may want to get a precision-attachment removable denture. It involves placing a crown on the adjacent tooth or teeth with a place for the attachment in the back so that no clasp shows. Removable bridges that contain precision attachments are usually made of gold-containing alloys combined with porcelain or acrylic teeth. Although considerably more costly than conventional removable bridges, precision-attachment removable bridges offer a much more esthetic result.

WHAT YOU SHOULD KNOW

PRECISION-ATTACHMENT REMOVABLE BRIDGE

ADVANTAGES

▶ Clasps are hidden

▶ Superior retention

DISADVANTAGES

▶ More expensive than conventional option

▶ Attachments can break and/or wear

▶ Involves more reduction of teeth

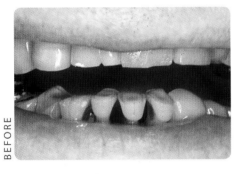
BEFORE

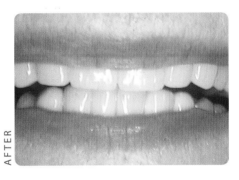
AFTER

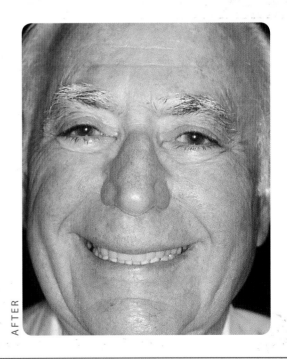
AFTER

To be precise » This 75-year-old president of a large corporation had worn down his upper and lower teeth. All of his remaining upper and lower teeth were crowned, and precision-attachment removable bridges were placed to rebuild his entire mouth. Notice how the longer front teeth look more youthful and handsome.

WHAT IS A COMPLETE DENTURE?

A complete denture is a removable prosthesis that replaces all of the teeth in an arch (upper or lower) as well as any missing supporting structures (gums and bone). The conventional complete denture is designed for patients who have lost all of their teeth or who need to have any remaining teeth extracted. The overdenture (a type of complete denture that fits over remaining teeth or implants) is also discussed in this section.

is A COMPLETE DENTURE RIGHT FOR ME?

Complete dentures offer an esthetic solution to patients who have lost all of their teeth. A complete denture may be the best option if you:

- Want to achieve a more youthful appearance
- Aren't a good candidate for implants
- Don't mind having to get it relined and eventually replaced
- Are looking for the most economical method of replacing all of your teeth

what to expect
COMPLETE DENTURE

The complete denture is a mixed blessing. On the one hand, it allows the dentist to change almost anything you want in your smile. On the other hand, after you lose your teeth the normal "landmarks" are gone—and so is the memory of how the teeth used to look. Be patient and work with a dentist who is willing to help you obtain the smile you desire. Also remember that dentures wear just as natural teeth do. If you want to keep your facial support and tone, your dentures will eventually need to be relined or remade.

6

Get a face lift without the surgery » When teeth are present and in good position, the lips and cheeks are properly supported. If the teeth are lost and not replaced, part of the facial tissue support also is lost. One of the primary advantages of the complete denture is its ability to maintain or even re-create lip and cheek support. Notice how much more youthful this woman's face is after placement of a well-made complete denture.

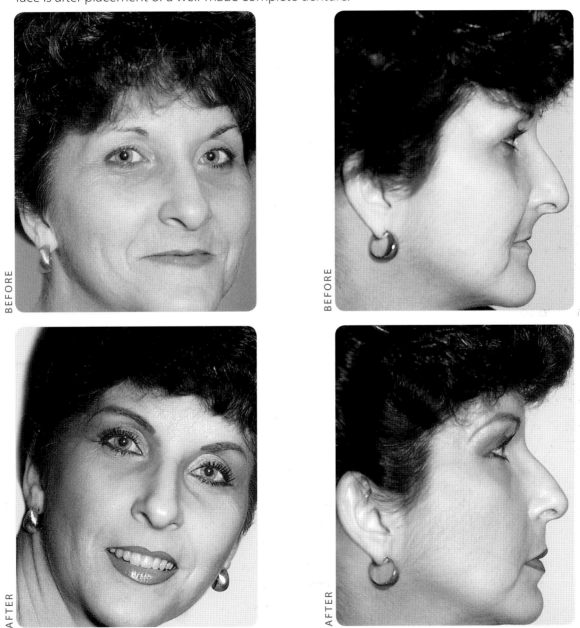

BEFORE

BEFORE

AFTER

AFTER

WHAT YOU SHOULD KNOW

OVERDENTURE

ADVANTAGES

▶ Can save roots

▶ Improves chewing ability

▶ Better fit and retention as compared to normal denture

▶ Less stress to supporting ridge tissue

▶ Provides a good transition to a full denture

▶ Allows the patient to retain some tactile sensation

DISADVANTAGES

▶ Attachment can break

▶ More costly than conventional denture

▶ May be slightly bulkier than fixed or removable partial dentures

smile 101 | What is an overdenture?

An overdenture, like a complete denture, is made to fit over the entire arch, but it is used for patients who still have teeth remaining that do not require extraction or who will have implants placed. The retained and reduced teeth or implants are used to help support the overdenture. Although this is a more expensive treatment option than a conventional complete denture, it provides considerable control over esthetics, a much stronger biting surface, and significantly greater retention.

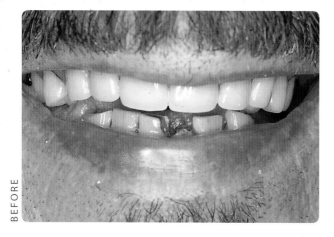

BEFORE

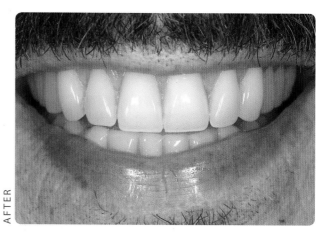

AFTER

Stay competitive with a young, healthy smile » This 66-year-old executive assistant needed a younger and healthier look to stay competitive in his industry. A new implant-retained overdenture was selected, which greatly helped denture retention and provided him the younger-looking smile he wanted.

6

what to eXpect

IMMEDIATE DENTURE

The procedure requires an initial office visit to make records. The laboratory then constructs a preliminary full denture that duplicates the appearance of your natural teeth or, if you want, improves them in color, form, and position. At the next appointment, your teeth can be removed and the immediate denture inserted. Because gum tissue will eventually shrink, however, a re-line or a new denture will be require in the future.

WHAT YOU SHOULD KNOW

LOSING A TOOTH

Don't assume that a tooth that's been knocked out can't be reimplanted. The directions below, provided by the American Association of Endodontists, outline the steps to be taken when a tooth is lost. Parents, teachers, and sports officials, in particular, should keep this information handy.

1. Remain calm while you try to locate the tooth.

2. Pick up the tooth gently, being careful to handle it by its crown, not by its roots.

3. Gently remove any debris from the tooth. Do not scrub or use any cleaning agents on the tooth.

4. Look for fractures in the roots. If there are no fractures, carefully replace the tooth in its socket or keep it moist in a glass of milk. There are also products available on the market that are specifically designed to keep a lost tooth moist. If neither of these are available, place the tooth in the mouth next to the cheek. Do not put the tooth in water!

5. See a dentist immediately, preferably within 30 minutes.

Solution 4 Implants

WHAT IS A DENTAL IMPLANT?

A dental implant is a metal or ceramic device that replaces the root of the natural tooth. After implants are placed in the bone, artificial teeth are attached to them, enabling normal function and natural tooth appearance. Whether an implant is right for you depends on where the implant will be placed, the kind and amount of bone available in your jaw, and the design of the restoration to be placed on the implant.

> **How It's Done**
> *see pages 228–230*

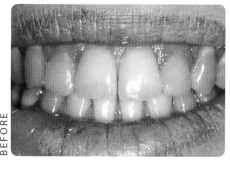

BEFORE

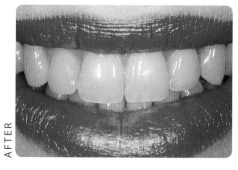

AFTER

As good as new » This patient fractured her upper left lateral incisor in an auto accident. The tooth was extracted and replaced with an implant, which was restored with a porcelain-bonded-to-metal crown. In addition, all of her teeth were bleached, and porcelain veneers were placed on her right lateral and both central incisors, giving the patient a beautiful and natural-looking smile.

expert tip Tired of loose dentures?

Patients with multiple missing teeth can also benefit from implant treatment if sufficient bone is present. Even if you have worn a fixed or removable bridge or a complete denture, you may still be a good candidate for implant dentistry. Implants act as an excellent source of anchorage for patients with loose or ill-fitting dentures.

6

FIND AN EXPERIENCED IMPLANT DENTIST

If you're considering dental implants, discuss all of your options with your dentist. Don't be afraid to ask questions and to seek a second opinion. Implant treatment is complex, and not all dentists perform it. Choose someone with experience; you want to receive the best care possible.

WHAT YOU SHOULD KNOW

HOME CARE IS IMPORTANT

Just because implants aren't "real" teeth doesn't mean oral hygiene is less important. Plaque accumulation on implants can cause inflammation of the gums and eventually loss of bone surrounding the teeth. Therefore, thorough cleaning twice a day is critical. Your dentist will discuss the best method for taking care of your particular implant.

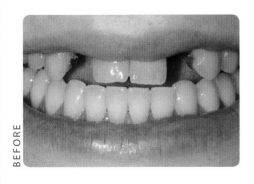 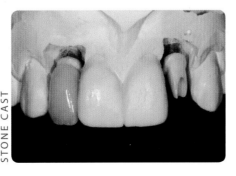 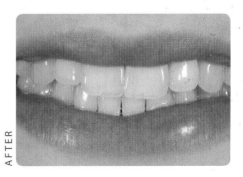

BEFORE STONE CAST AFTER

The beauty of implants » This patient lost two lateral incisors but did not want to wear a fixed bridge to replace them. The center image shows the zirconia abutments and one of the final crowns on the stone cast. Note how natural the smile looks with the two final crowns on the implants plus four porcelain veneers on the central incisors and canines.

WHICH SOLUTION IS BEST FOR **YOU?**

FIXED BRIDGE	REMOVABLE BRIDGE
TREATMENT TIME	
2–4 weeks	2–4 office visits
MAINTENANCE	
Clean daily under the bridge with floss threaders.	• *Conventional:* Remove and clean after eating. • *Precision-attachment:* Clean and adjust regularly.
RESULTS	
Esthetic tooth replacement	• *Conventional:* Least expensive way to replace missing teeth • *Precision-attachment:* More esthetic than a conventional removable bridge
TREATMENT LONGEVITY*	
Conventional and cantilever: 5–15 years *Resin-bonded:* 5–10 years	5–10 years
COST†	
• *Conventional and cantilever:* $950 to $3,500 per tooth • *Resin-bonded:* $650 to $2,500 per tooth	• *Conventional:* $850 to $3,500 per tooth, depending on the design and material used • *Precision-attachment:* $950 to $5,000 per tooth
ADVANTAGES	
• Feels more like natural teeth • Can be most esthetic • Helps prevent movement of adjacent and opposing teeth • Improves the bite • *Resin-bonded:* Avoids reduction of adjacent teeth	• Economical method of tooth replacement • Easy to repair
DISADVANTAGES	
• If one of the attached teeth fails, the entire bridge fails. • May be difficult to repair if porcelain chips or fractures. • Requires an anesthetic.	• Can cause wear and trauma to attached teeth • May not be as esthetic as a fixed bridge • *Precision-attachment:* Attachments can break or wear

*This estimate is based on the author's clinical experience combined with three university research studies and insurance company estimates. Your own experience could be different, depending on many factors, only some of which you and your dentist can control.

†Fees will vary from dentist to dentist based on the difficulty of the procedure, patient problems, patient dental and medical history, expectations, and dentist qualifications, including technical and artistic expertise.

‡Expect to pay extra for esthetic temporaries.

6

COMPLETE DENTURE	IMPLANTS
2–5 office visits	• *Surgical placement:* about 1 hour per implant • *Healing:* about 3 mo in lower jaw and 6 mo in upper jaw • *Second surgery (if needed):* 30–60 min • *Immediate loading:* 2 hours or more per implant
Clean after meals to remove and prevent stains on denture.	• Floss and perform home care daily. • Have a restorative exam every 3–4 mo.
Esthetically pleasing results are possible	• Natural appearance possible • Good individual functioning
5–10 years; tooth fracture may occur (but is easy to repair), and relining may be necessary during this time	Indefinite, barring infection. Life expectancy of the restoration is the same as described elsewhere (for a crown, 5–15 years)
$525 to $5,000 per denture (expect to pay up to 2×–3× this amount for special "cosmetic" dentures)	$985 to $2,800 per implant (plus additional cost of crowns)
• Excellent esthetics possible • More youthful appearance obtainable • Supports lips and cheeks • Can improve speech	• Most closely approximate having your own natural teeth • Avoid reduction of adjacent teeth • Can be flossed like natural teeth • Help preserve bone • Have approximately 95% success rate over 40-year life span of implant
• Less chewing efficiency. • Retention may be a problem. • Needs maintenance. • May need to be replaced every 5–10 years. • May impede speech in some instances.	• 3%–7% failure rate. • Ceramic implants can fracture. • Abutment screws can loosen or break. • Requires an anesthetic.

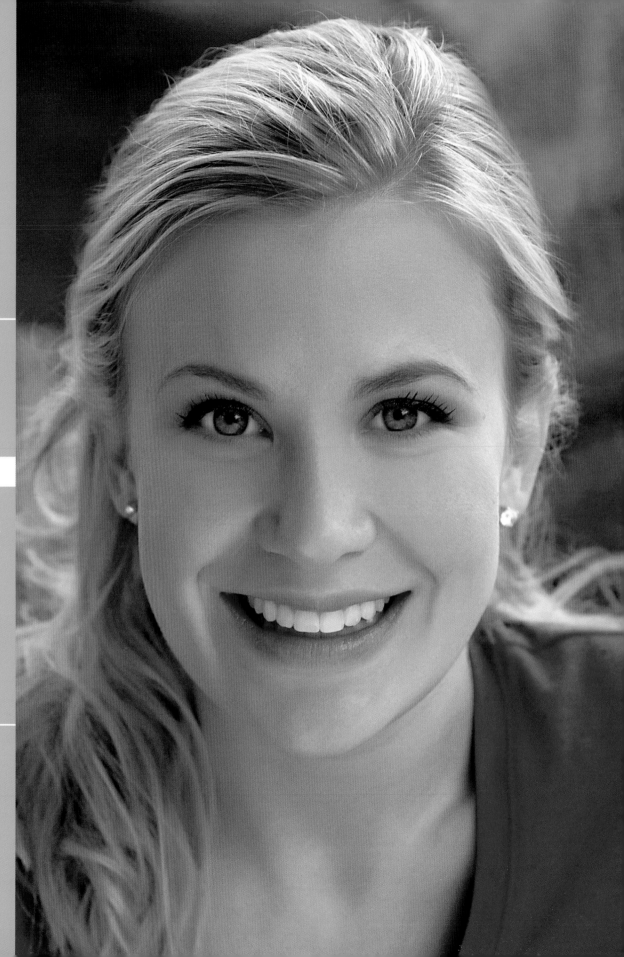

7

Straighten up and Smile Right

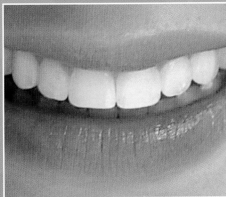

There is no reason to go through life with a crooked smile.

Living with anything less than beautiful, straight white teeth can be a source of great unhappiness. If you have crowded or crooked teeth that overlap, protrude, or recede in a haphazard fashion, this chapter will tell you how you can achieve a new, gorgeous smile.

Although orthodontics is most often the best way to correct crowded teeth, it is not the only way. Less expensive and less time-consuming methods may be used if the problem is not too severe. Although the teeth may not be in perfect alignment, creating the illusion that they are may allow you to achieve your esthetic goal.

Crowded or crooked teeth may require a combination of techniques described in this chapter. Your ideal treatment, for example, may include orthodontics to reposition the teeth followed by bonding, veneers, or crowns to improve esthetics. The choice of treatment ultimately depends upon your commitment of time and money, as well as your dental and esthetic needs.

Solution 1 Cosmetic Contouring

NEED AN ESTHETIC QUICK FIX?

Cosmetic contouring is a simple and painless reshaping procedure in which tooth structure is contoured with finely ground diamonds. It's used to improve the appearance of the teeth by giving the illusion of uniformity and alignment.

IS COSMETIC CONTOURING RIGHT FOR ME?

Although its simplicity generally makes it the most preferred therapy, cosmetic contouring is not right for everyone. Cosmetic contouring may be the best option if you:

- Have only slightly crowded teeth
- Do not wish to have an anesthetic administered
- Prefer a relatively inexpensive and quick procedure
- Agree with a compromise solution

Straighter teeth in an hour » This television producer wanted to improve her smile without wearing braces. A 1-hour appointment was all it took to help create an illusion of straight teeth and a new smile.

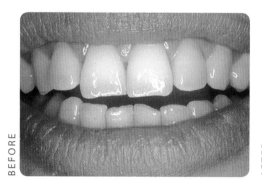

BEFORE

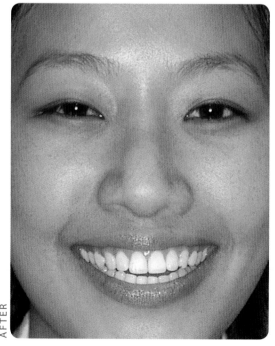

AFTER

7

104

WHAT YOU SHOULD KNOW

BEFORE SELECTING COSMETIC CONTOURING

▶ Your dentist should evaluate the effect contouring may have on your teeth. Your bite must continue to be correct if the health of the teeth, as well as the proper distribution of pressure during normal oral functioning, is to be maintained.

▶ The thickness of the tooth enamel must be checked. The removal of too much enamel can expose the dentin, resulting in discoloration and possibly sensitivity.

▶ A conflict may arise between maintaining optimum function and achieving maximum esthetics. In these cases, the final decision should be based on a trade-off among esthetics, the degree of bite change, and the health of the teeth.

▶ A plaster cast may be constructed so that you can see the limitations in your particular case.

▶ Cosmetic contouring should not be performed on children's teeth. It can cause slight sensitivity—not only during the procedure, but afterward—because they have a larger amount of sensitive pulp tissue.

A straight smile is a happy smile! » This executive assistant was unhappy with her crooked, worn, and chipped teeth. Although orthodontic treatment would have been an ideal option, she chose cosmetic contouring. This 1-hour painless procedure was all it took to reshape the teeth and create an illusion of straightness. In one carefully planned appointment her old smile was transformed into a new happy smile that matches her cheerful personality.

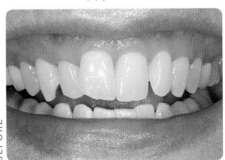

BEFORE

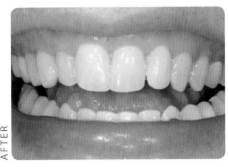

AFTER

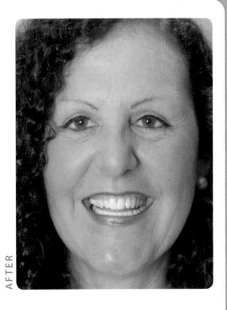

AFTER

Solution 2 Bonding

DOES YOUR SMILE NEED A LITTLE SOMETHING MORE?

If cosmetic contouring alone cannot shape up your smile, it can be combined with composite resin bonding to "build out" the fronts or backs of the teeth to fall in line with neighboring teeth. The result is an illusion of straightness that can be quite pleasing.

▷ How It's Done
see page 217

smile 101 Can lower teeth be bonded?

Your bite may be a limiting factor in the success of bonding the lower front teeth. However, it's sometimes possible to reduce the amount of stress on the lower teeth by altering the way in which the upper teeth contact them.

expert tip Braces may be best!

If your crowded teeth are causing a narrow or constricted arch, consider orthodontics. If this isn't feasible, however, a combined treatment consisting of cosmetic contouring and bonding may help correct arch malalignment.

A beautiful smile with no braces » This patient was displeased with her crowded teeth but didn't want orthodontic treatment of any kind. Although several dentists had refused to provide any treatment other than orthodontics, this attractive new smile was conservatively accomplished in two appointments involving a wax-up, some artistic cosmetic contouring, and composite resin bonding.

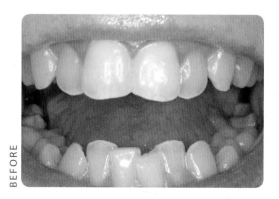

BEFORE

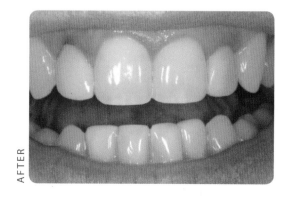

AFTER

Getting rid of overlap » This 30-year-old woman disliked her overlapping front teeth. The two upper front teeth were cosmetically contoured to look narrower and to reduce some of the overlap. The adjacent lateral incisors were then built out with composite resin to blend in with the newly contoured central incisors. This helped to round out the arch, making the teeth look much straighter. The entire procedure was done in one appointment without an anesthetic.

BEFORE

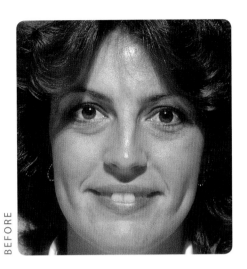

AFTER

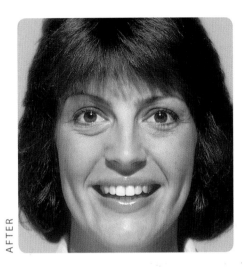

expert tip **Lighten up!**

Bonding also may be used to lighten crowded teeth. However, if not all of the teeth are to be bonded, the adjacent teeth should be bleached before bonding is performed. Otherwise, some teeth will be much lighter than others—not an esthetically pleasing result!

BEFORE

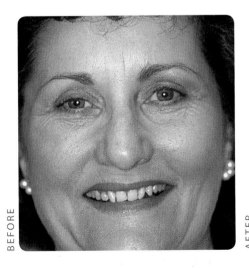

AFTER

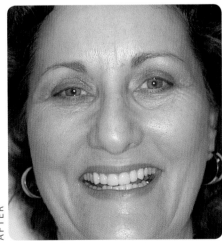

Keeping things in proportion » This patient had lateral incisors that overlapped her central incisors, which not only destroyed proportion in her smile but also created spaces. In addition, she had a retained baby tooth. The teeth were contoured slightly to improve their proportion, then composite resin was placed directly on the front teeth. Note the improvement in tooth size and form that was achieved with this one-appointment procedure.

Solution 3 Porcelain Veneers

In many cases, porcelain veneers can also provide a reasonable compromise when you want to avoid orthodontic treatment. Crooked and crowded teeth laminated with porcelain veneers will usually give the result of a polished, natural-looking smile.

▷ ┤ How It's Done
    see pages 218–219

Straighter teeth—No braces required » This internationally known tennis personality wanted to improve his smile. The before photo (from a commercial advertisement, courtesy of Swatch, Inc) shows crowded, disproportionate teeth as well as a high lip line. The final result, achieved through conservative gum surgery combined with porcelain veneers, shows a more handsome face with teeth that are more proportionate for his face.

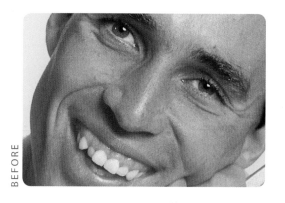
BEFORE

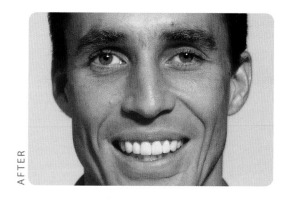
AFTER

A conservative way to restore crooked teeth » This woman was unhappy with her crowded and discolored teeth as well as her old silver fillings. She didn't want to invest the time in orthodontic treatment and wanted to preserve as much of her tooth structure as possible. Porcelain veneers plus a special technique called porcelain laminate overlays, which cover both the front and top of a tooth, were used to achieve the goal of a conservative, quick, and esthetic solution.

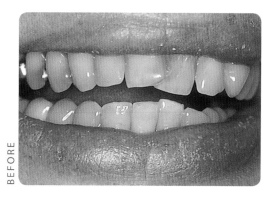
BEFORE

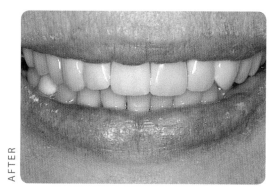
AFTER

7

Solution 4 Crowns

Getting it straight » Crowded and discolored upper teeth and spaces between the lower teeth spoiled the smile of this 38-year-old business owner. Although orthodontics was suggested as the ideal treatment, he chose a compromise that consisted of bonding the lower teeth and crowning the upper teeth. The final result is a much more pleasing smile.

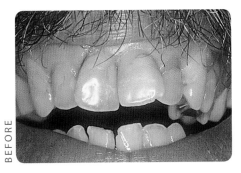

BEFORE

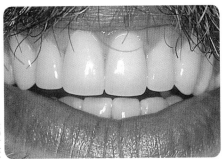

AFTER

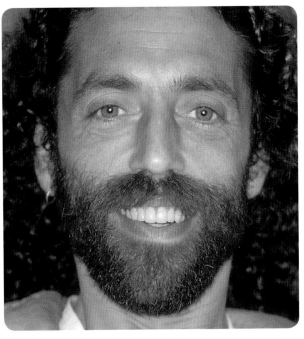

AFTER

LOOKING FOR DRAMATIC RESULTS?

Crowns are another way to correct the problem of crowded teeth. Although they may be more costly and time-consuming than most of the previously discussed cosmetic procedures, they can produce a more dramatic change and may be a preferable alternative, particularly when teeth are erupting, damaged, or receding at extreme angles from the root structure.

> How It's Done
see pages 220–225

A good case for crowns » This 58-year-old attorney was not happy with her crowded and discolored teeth. She also had worn down some of her anterior teeth, producing a reverse smile line. A much straighter and younger-looking smile was created with all-ceramic crowns.

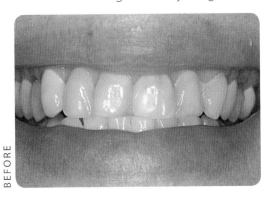

BEFORE

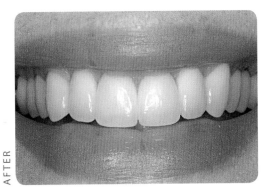

AFTER

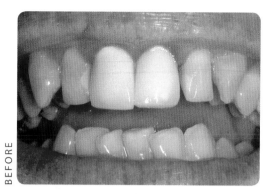

BEFORE

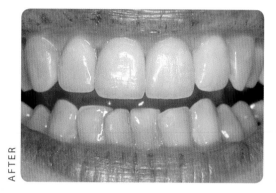

AFTER

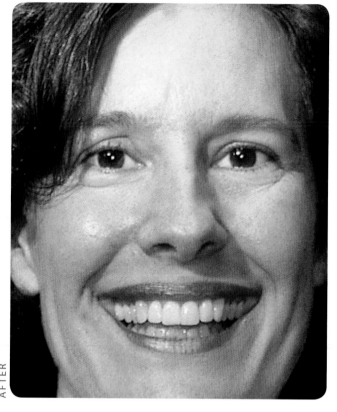

AFTER

Take an integrated approach » A previous dentist had difficulty making appropriately sized crowns for this patient's front teeth due to crowding. By reducing the adjacent teeth for porcelain veneers, plus slimming the width of the canines, it was possible to crown only the two central incisors to improve the smile line. Porcelain veneers were placed on the two lateral incisors, and the canines were bonded with composite resin. The final result shows a pretty smile that now complements her face.

expert tip Look before you leap!

If you think you may want to crown your crooked teeth, it's wise to spend a little extra money for a wax-up or trial smile. This will allow you to see the intended result before your natural teeth are prepared. You can make a serious mistake by crowning crooked teeth and thinking they will look terrific. You may not be happy with the result since the final crowns may be much thinner than your own teeth. In such cases, you will not only have lost the money spent on crowns, but you will probably end up undergoing the treatment you should have gotten in the first place—orthodontics.

7

WHAT YOU SHOULD KNOW

CHOOSE CROWNS WITH CAUTION

Crowns have limited use for crowded and crooked teeth because the orientation of the teeth to be crowned must be aligned with the surrounding teeth. If they aren't, the crowns won't be able to compensate for the difference. In other words, the same problem that existed with the natural teeth may also exist with the crowns.

Tooth size is another major factor to consider because each tooth needs to be—or at least appear to be—proportional. The more teeth that are treated, the less obvious any distortions will be. If only one or two teeth are crowned, however, there may be a noticeable difference between the crowned teeth and the natural ones, depending on the space involved. Careful cosmetic contouring of both the teeth to be crowned and the adjacent teeth may make the final result appear more harmonious in size.

Solution 5 Orthodontics

BRACE YOURSELF!

Orthodontics is the treatment of choice when the top priority is keeping the teeth natural and unaltered. It is, without a doubt, the best way to correct malpositioned or crooked teeth. With orthodontic treatment, the teeth eventually will become aligned proportionally, making it your safest bet for a long-lasting, economical, and esthetic solution.

> How It's Done
> *see page 231*

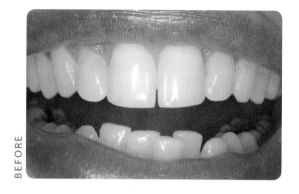

BEFORE

Invisible braces: A clear solution for crooked teeth » This beautiful 50-year-old makeup artist was unhappy with her crowded lower front teeth. In a matter of months the teeth were straightened using clear plastic matrices. The procedure was painless, and no one noticed she was having her teeth straightened.

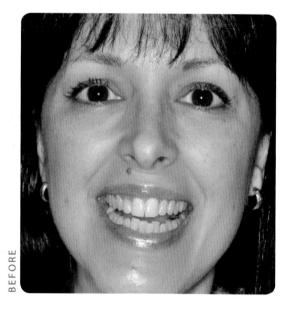

BEFORE

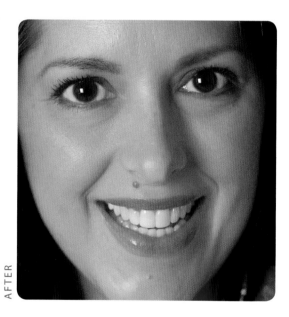

AFTER

smile 101 Think you're too old for braces?

More than 20% of the patients now seen by orthodontists are adults, many of whom are more than 50 years old!

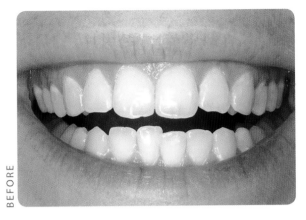

BEFORE

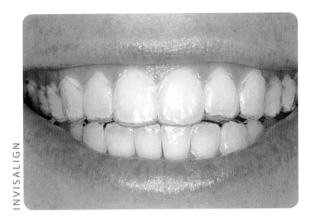

INVISALIGN

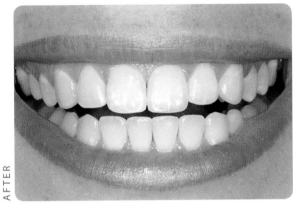

AFTER

Time for realignment? » Although this woman had orthodontics when she was a young girl, she failed to wear her retainers, and the teeth began to crowd again. The patient chose to use Invisalign to realign her teeth quickly and discreetly. It only took 4 months to straighten her teeth, which were then reshaped using cosmetic contouring to eliminate the chips and effects of wear. The result is a new smile with long-lasting beauty.

WHAT YOU SHOULD KNOW

ORTHODONTICS HAS COME A LONG WAY

In years past, orthodontics was shunned by many adults because treatment was lengthy, and traditional metal braces were conspicuous and unattractive. Now dentistry has seen the advent of tooth-colored brackets, lingual ("behind the teeth") braces, and removable appliances. The newest orthodontic treatment is "invisible" braces (such as Invisalign), a series of clear, removable, transparent matrices that are changed every 2 weeks. Each matrix moves the teeth to a specific position according to the custom computerized plan until the ideal placement is achieved. Most minor crowding can be corrected in 4 to 12 months, while more complex problems can be resolved in 18 to 30 months. However, compliance in wearing the appliance approximately 22 hours a day is mandatory. Invisible braces are easy to maintain with proper home hygiene and require less time in the dentist's chair since there are no wires or brackets to replace, making them a great option for adults. An added benefit is that, if advised by your dentist, you can place bleaching gel inside the matrices and bleach your teeth at the same time you are straightening them.

113

what to eXpect

EXTRACTION MAY BE REQUIRED

Occasionally, the orthodontist may recommend that a tooth or teeth be extracted prior to realigning the teeth to make space, particularly in cases where crowding is causing bone loss between the teeth.

BEFORE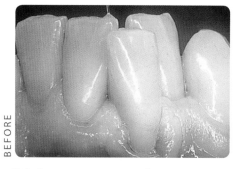

ORTHODONTICS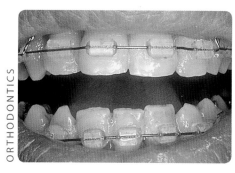

AFTER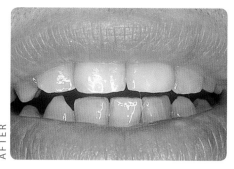

Make some room! » This 36-year-old salesman noticed his front teeth becoming more crowded as he aged. The protruding lower front tooth was extracted, and the remaining teeth were repositioned with tooth-colored brackets. It took less than 12 months to produce the results seen here.

BEFORE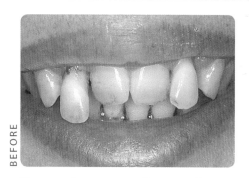

ORTHODONTICS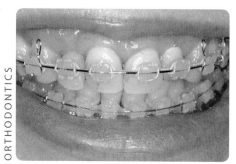

AFTER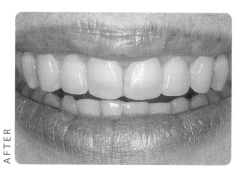

Get a picture-perfect smile » No matter how bad your teeth look, there are always treatment options that can help you achieve a beautiful smile. This 48-year-old woman had crowded teeth combined with periodontal disease and missing teeth. Treatment consisted of removal of her two lateral incisors followed by orthodontics, placement of two implants with crowns in the site of her upper posterior teeth, and two resin-bonded bridges to replace the missing laterals. Although it took several years, she now has a smile that matches her good looks.

7

Put your teeth in their place » Severe crowding and the discolored front teeth of this businesswoman ruined an otherwise attractive face. At first glance, one may think that crowning the teeth would produce an instant esthetic result; however, it wouldn't correct the severity of the angle of protrusion. With crowning alone, the teeth would look better, but would still stick out too far. Thus, orthodontics was the first step. The teeth were repositioned so that each would have proper space, then four crowns were placed. Note the relaxed muscle tissue and especially the improvement in the upper lip in relation to the teeth. Worn and discolored teeth age a smile—this woman looks much younger with a brighter new smile.

BEFORE

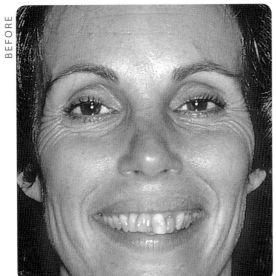

ORTHODONTICS

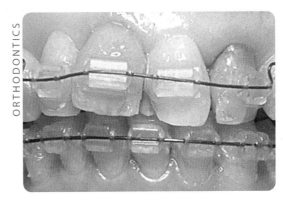

BEFORE

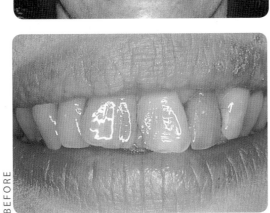

AFTER

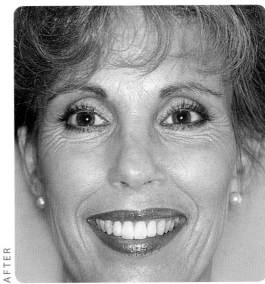

WHICH SOLUTION IS BEST FOR **YOU?**

	COSMETIC CONTOURING	BONDING
TREATMENT TIME	About 1 hour or less	1–2 hours per tooth
MAINTENANCE	Brush and floss daily.	• Have a professional cleaning 3–4 times per year. • Eat wisely—bonded teeth can chip more easily than your enamel. • Push floss in and pull it through teeth rather than popping it out. • See dentist for repair as necessary.
RESULTS	Immediate reshaping of tooth structure, making crowded teeth appear to be the appropriate size and straighter	Straighter teeth in 1 office visit
TREATMENT LONGEVITY[*]	Indefinite	5–8 years
COST[†]	$350 to $2,500 per arch	$175 to $1,500 per tooth (repairs may cost $145 to $485)
ADVANTAGES	• Less expensive than other forms of esthetic treatment • Permanent results • Immediate correction • Minimum treatment time • Generally painless; no anesthetic required	• Conservative (little or no tooth reduction). • Sometimes reversible. • Less expensive than veneers or crowns. • No anesthetic required. • Teeth appear and feel straighter.
DISADVANTAGES	• Does not reposition teeth. • Improvement may be limited by functional considerations. • Can cause discomfort for children with large pulp canals. • Does not improve color.	• Does not reposition teeth. • Does not address gum inflammation due to crowding. • Can stain or chip more easily than veneers or crowns. • May require frequent repair. • Teeth may appear and feel thicker.

[*]This estimate is based on the author's clinical experience combined with three university research studies and insurance company estimates. Your own experience could be different, depending on many factors, only some of which you and your dentist can control.

[†]Fees will vary from dentist to dentist based on the difficulty of the procedure, patient problems, patient dental and medical history, expectations, and dentist qualifications, including technical and artistic expertise.

[‡]Expect to pay extra for esthetic temporaries.

7

PORCELAIN VENEERS	CROWNS	ORTHODONTICS
2 office visits; 1–4 hours each (more time needed for more extensive treatment)	2 office visits; 1–4 hours each for up to 4 teeth (more time needed for additional teeth or more extensive treatment)	6–30 months, depending on amount of crowding and method selected
• Have a professional cleaning 3–4 times per year. • Take special care when biting into or chewing hard foods. • Get yearly fluoride treatments. • Brush and floss daily. • Use a fluoride toothpaste and mouthwash as prescribed by your dentist.	• Avoid biting down on hard foods and ice. • Get yearly fluoride treatments. • Brush and floss daily. • Use a fluoride toothpaste and mouthwash as prescribed by your dentist.	• Brush and floss daily with special care. • Have a professional cleaning 3–4 times per year. • Schedule adjustment checkups every 3–4 weeks during treatment. • Wear retainers indefinitely, at least a few nights per week.
A polished, natural-appearing result that can make teeth seem straighter and is more stain resistant than bonding	The best esthetic results in terms of reshaping teeth	Crowded and overlapping teeth can be straightened
5–12 years	5–15 years (directly related to fractures, problems with tissues, and decay)	Generally permanent if retainer is worn at least a few nights per week
$950 to $3,500 per tooth[‡]	$950 to $3,500 per tooth[‡]	$1,500 to $7,500, depending on the number of teeth involved and the appliance used; lingual braces may cost up to $2,000 more per arch
• Less wear and chipping than bonding. • Excellent bond to enamel. • Minimal staining and loss of color or luster. • More proportional results due to lab construction. • Long-lasting results. • Gum tissue tolerates porcelain well.	• Teeth can be lightened to any shade. • Less time required than orthodontics. • Less staining than bonding. • Last longer than bonding or veneers. • Offer greatest opportunity to improve tooth form.	• Straightens misaligned teeth • Permanent results for most people if retainers are worn • Little or no tooth reduction required • Usually less expensive than veneers, crowns, or bonding, depending on number of teeth involved • Improved tissue health due to better cleaning access following treatment
• More expensive than bonding. • Difficult to repair if the veneer cracks or chips. • Margins may "wash out" and require repair.	• Can fracture • Require an anesthetic • Not a permanent solution • More expensive than contouring or bonding • Irreversible • Can trigger pulp irritation • Can induce tooth sensitivity for a short time	• Time consuming. • Teeth may return to original position if retainers are not worn. • May take a few weeks to get used to appliances. • May be temporarily unesthetic in appearance. • Brackets can irritate soft tissue. • Thorough cleanings are more difficult during treatment.

8

FIND OUT . . .

WHAT TYPE OF BITE
YOU HAVE

WHICH TREATMENT OPTIONS
ARE BEST FOR YOUR BITE

HOW LENGTHENING
YOUR FRONT TEETH MAY
IMPROVE YOUR SMILE

Finding Closure

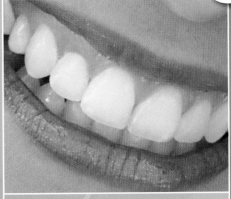

Don't let a bad bite ruin your sexy smile.

The teeth and bone structure form the foundation of the mouth and its surrounding tissues. When this framework isn't aligned, a malocclusion (or bad bite) results. On the surface, this often appears as little more than an esthetic problem, but the ramifications of improperly aligned teeth are more far-reaching. Bad bites can cause problems ranging from headaches to faulty hearing. They also can cause digestive problems that affect overall health, not to mention disposition.

Many adults, as well as children, suffer from bite disorders that affect their physical and social well-being. Fortunately, modern dentistry offers a variety of ways to treat improperly aligned bites—many of which are imperceptible to others. This chapter outlines various bite disorders and the options that are available to treat them.

WHAT
CAUSES BAD BITES?

A bad bite is typically caused by genetics. For example, the teeth may not fit in the jaws properly, or the teeth may not be in a correct relationship with the rest of the face. Destructive habits, such as lip or nail biting or clenching and grinding teeth, also can cause bad bites. Finally, loss of teeth without proper replacement can cause the bite and the face to collapse, resulting in an aged and unattractive appearance.

expert tip Don't wait to replace missing teeth!

When a tooth is missing due to loss or extraction, other teeth will shift. This can cause a variety of bite and gum problems that can be expensive and time-consuming to correct. It is wise, therefore, to replace missing teeth as quickly as possible. See chapter 6 for more information.

Bring your grinding to a halt » This 28-year-old computer expert had excessive abrasion caused by bruxism (grinding of the teeth), which led to erosion of the enamel on the biting edges of the lower teeth. The eroded and stained areas were restored with composite resin bonding, and cosmetic contouring was performed to blend the shapes and improve the smile line.

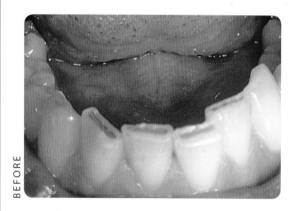

BEFORE

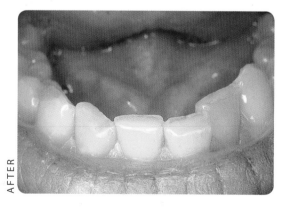

AFTER

what to eXpect

MOUTH APPLIANCES

- Often suggested for patients experiencing bruxism or a temporomandibular disorder (TMD).

- Prevent tooth wear and loss and can alleviate head, neck, ear, or back pain.

- May be adjusted over time to improve and rebalance your bite. It also may be necessary to rebuild your teeth so that they fit this new position and the muscles operate correctly and comfortably.

- Treatment lasts 3 months to 1 year for most patients but may continue indefinitely for certain problems.

- Must be worn either nightly or full time for a specified period.

- Cost $850 to $5,000, depending on amount and frequency of treatment.

What is bruxism?

Bruxism is involuntary grinding or clenching of the teeth. It usually leads to tooth wear, which can contribute to bite problems and TMDs as well as esthetic problems. Worn teeth become smaller and are usually darker in color, creating an aged look.

In severe cases, consider surgery!

Orthognathic surgery is sometimes the ideal solution for severe bite problems, especially when facial distortion is a concern. It is often used in combination with orthodontics to put the jaws in a more ideal relationship, thereby shortening the time of treatment and helping to achieve a more esthetic result. Orthognathic surgery is covered in more detail in chapter 11.

BAD BITES AND THE TEMPOROMANDIBULAR JOINT

When the teeth are out of alignment, the facial muscles may spasm, creating misalignment of the jaw. This can lead to temporomandibular joint (TMJ) disorders, also called TMDs. Symptoms can include headaches, neck pain, back pain, and earaches. Treatment of TMDs depends on the severity of the disorder and ranges from muscle relaxation therapy to orthognathic surgery. No cosmetic procedures should be performed until the TMD is corrected.

WHAT YOU SHOULD KNOW

IS YOUR NEW BITE A BAD BITE?

Occasionally, even properly constructed restorations can contribute to bite problems. This typically occurs when a disharmony already exists in the mouth. In such cases, any irritation or change—even as minor as that caused by crowns or orthodontics—can initiate a muscle spasm and TMJ disturbance. Such problems may be unforeseen by dentists. When noted, however, they should be corrected quickly. If allowed to persist, they can be extremely difficult to repair.

There are several different kinds of bite disorders, and their severity can vary widely from person to person. This section explains and illustrates each of the most common bite problems and presents a chart that compares treatment options to help you determine which one may be best for you.

DOES **THIS** LOOK LIKE YOUR BITE?

Each of these illustrations gives a typical example of the bite problems described in this chapter. If one of these looks like your bite, turn to the related section to see what alternatives you have for better function and esthetics.

DEEP OVERBITE

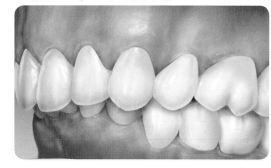

CLOSED BITE

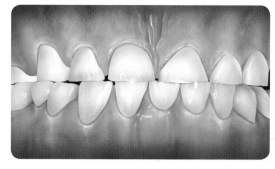

CROSSBITE

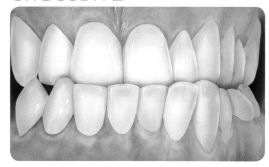

OPEN BITE

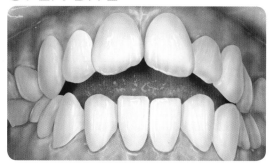

PROTRUSION

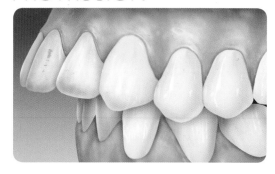

Deep Overbite

WHAT IS THE **BEST** TREATMENT?

The treatment of choice for deep overbite is orthodontics, which may be combined with orthognathic surgery depending on the severity of the problem. Orthodontic treatment may consist of intruding the anterior teeth, erupting the posterior teeth, or a combination of both, based on your facial profile and growth potential, as well as the extent of the overbite.

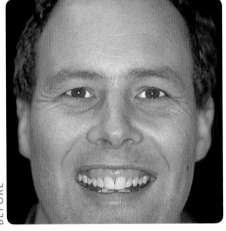

BEFORE

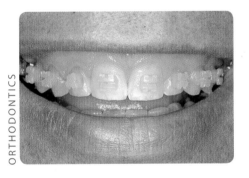

ORTHODONTICS

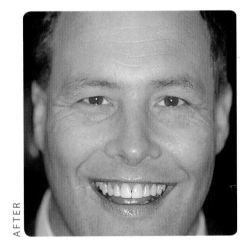

AFTER

Changing your bite can improve your whole look » This dentist was not happy with his gummy smile and worn teeth, which resulted from a deep overbite. Treatment took approximately 2 years and consisted of orthodontics followed by cosmetic gum surgery and bleaching. This experience not only gave the dentist the smile he wanted but also helped him relate to patients who wanted to improve their own smiles.

WHAT IS DEEP OVERBITE?

One of the bite problems that is most detrimental to facial esthetics is the deep overbite, which is almost complete overlap of the upper front teeth over the lower front teeth. The edges of the lower teeth may actually bite into the gum tissue of the upper palate.

Closed Bite

WHAT IS CLOSED BITE?

Some tooth wear is a natural function of aging. As long as it doesn't change your bite, it isn't a functional problem. Occasionally, however, tooth wear causes a closed bite, which can be a serious disorder. For example, extreme wear of the tooth structure in the back of the mouth can cause partial disintegration of the lower facial tissue. It can give you an aged appearance—as if you have no teeth. This problem can exist even in young people.

WHAT IS THE BEST TREATMENT?

If the closed bite is not too severe, the back teeth often can be built up with crowns or onlays (see pages 52–53), which allows the front teeth to be lengthened through bonding, veneers, or crowns. However, opening the bite through orthodontic treatment is typically the best option. Restorative procedures such as bridges, bonding, or veneers can be performed after the orthodontic treatment is complete. Orthognathic surgery also may be required if the lower jaw needs to be repositioned.

Tooth wear can lead to a closed bite » This 30-year-old salesman complained of unattractive teeth. His habits of clenching and bruxism had caused considerable tooth wear. He was also missing all the teeth behind the left canine, which caused bite collapse in the back, lip sag, and a tense look in his face. Treatment for this patient consisted of wearing a removable plastic bite appliance for 3 months to open the jaws slightly to the original bite position, followed by placement of fixed bridges and full crowns. Note how the new crowns and improved bite relationship helped produce a more relaxed lip line.

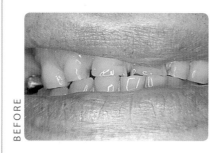

BEFORE

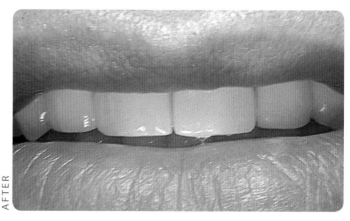

AFTER

Crossbite

WHAT IS THE **BEST** TREATMENT?

Although full crowns or composite resin bonding often can be used to "build out" the upper arch, this treatment achieves only limited esthetic modification. The best way to correct a crossbite is through orthodontics. If the crossbite is particularly severe, orthognathic surgery may be required in addition to orthodontics. This combined approach can result in a dramatic improvement in facial appearance. Best of all, the teeth tend to remain in their new positions once the condition is corrected.

Get an early start for best results » This young boy had a crossbite in which the upper front teeth closed behind his lower teeth. The best treatment for this condition is orthodontics. The first of a two-phase orthodontic treatment plan was aimed at facial development. The second phase occurred during his teen years and involved the use of tooth-colored porcelain braces to help align his teeth. Fortunately for this young man, the treatment was started early enough to help his face develop normally and to guide his teeth into a good alignment, helping to produce a great smile.

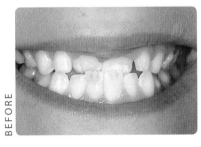

BEFORE

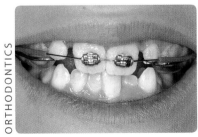

ORTHODONTICS

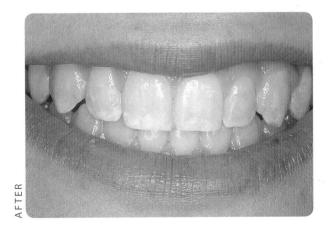

AFTER

WHAT IS CROSSBITE?

In a normal bite, the upper teeth slightly overlap the lower teeth. A crossbite results when the opposite occurs: when the lower teeth overlap the upper teeth. It can occur in both the front and back teeth. When a crossbite develops in the front teeth, one result is a protruding chin.

Open Bite

WHAT IS OPEN BITE?

Occasionally, the upper and lower front teeth cannot come together when the back teeth are touching. This condition is commonly referred to as an open bite. Heredity, as well as habits such as tongue thrusting, thumb sucking, and pencil biting, can cause open bites. Although people with open bites aren't always aware of the problem, one telltale symptom is difficulty biting with the front teeth. In addition, open bites cause protrusion of the upper lip, making it difficult for patients with open bites to close their lips over their teeth without straining.

WHAT IS THE BEST TREATMENT?

Orthodontics, occasionally combined with orthognathic surgery, is the best treatment for an open bite. It not only corrects tooth deformity but also moves underlying bone inward, enabling the lips to close properly.

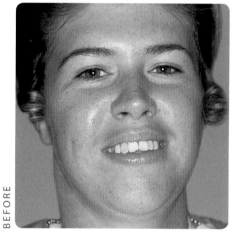

BEFORE

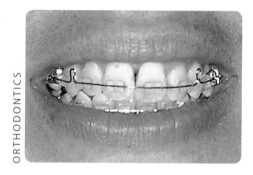

ORTHODONTICS

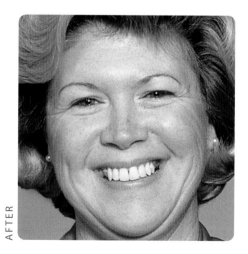

AFTER

Long-lasting solution for open bite » This woman was disturbed by the esthetic and functional problems created by her open bite. It was virtually impossible for her lips to close over the teeth without muscle strain, and it was difficult for her to bite into foods with her front teeth. Orthodontic treatment corrected the open bite, placing the teeth in a more normal relationship. A more feminine smile is the result of the new tooth position.

Protrusion

WHAT IS THE **BEST** TREATMENT?

Orthodontic treatment, combined with orthognathic surgery in severe cases, is the best way to correct protrusion. In some cases, two to four teeth may be extracted to achieve good results. Keep in mind, however, that overcorrection is a major concern when teeth are extracted. Overcorrection occurs when the teeth are moved back too far, resulting in a sunken-in appearance. No matter how severe your protrusion, do not have your upper teeth extracted and replaced with a bridge. This typically won't correct the bone deformity and may seriously impair your chewing ability.

WHAT IS PROTRUSION?

Protruded upper front teeth, often called "buck teeth," can detract from even the best of smiles. In severe cases, protrusion results in facial deformity and an inability to close the lips over the teeth.

Immediate results for protruding teeth » This prima ballerina was concerned about her protruding and discolored teeth. Although orthodontic treatment would have been the ideal solution, she opted for immediate results with composite resin bonding of the upper and lower front teeth. Two appointments were all it took to achieve this attractive result. Although the protrusion still exists, the teeth look much better. The smile now becomes an important part of this beautiful face.

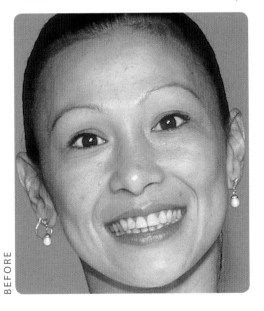

BEFORE

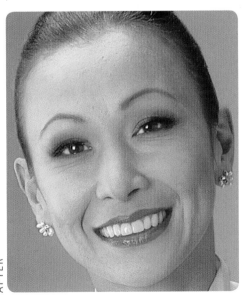

AFTER

WHICH SOLUTION IS BEST FOR **YOUR** BITE?

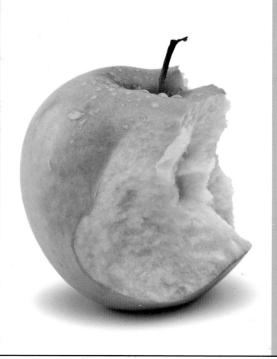

ORTHODONTICS	COSMETIC CONTOURING
DEEP OVERBITE OR CLOSED BITE	
Advantages • Best option to correct deep overbite • Longest lasting • Can help cure or prevent TMJ pain • Can prevent excessive wear if treated early enough *Disadvantages* • Takes 6–24 mo • Usually requires wearing a retainer indefinitely	*Advantages* • Good for esthetically shaping the teeth as a final touch • Completed in 1 office visit *Disadvantages* • Does not correct the problem
CROSSBITE	
Advantages • Most effective • Longest lasting *Disadvantages* • Takes 4–6 mo if only 1 or 2 teeth are involved • Requires 6–24 mo if more than 2 teeth are involved • May need to be combined with orthognathic surgery	*Advantages* • Can reshape teeth in opposite arch to help improve bite • Completed in 1 office visit • Long lasting • Inexpensive *Disadvantages* • Does not correct the problem
OPEN BITE	
Advantages • Improves ability to bite. • Can improve lip position and esthetics. • Can be combined with orthognathic surgery to reduce treatment time and improve facial results. *Disadvantages* • Time consuming. • Retention may be a problem depending on severity of bite problem and habits. • Usually requires wearing a retainer indefinitely.	*Advantages* • Good for esthetically shaping the teeth as a final touch • Completed in 1 office visit *Disadvantages* • Does not correct the problem
PROTRUSION	
Advantages • Most effective. • Longest lasting. • Can be combined with orthognathic surgery in severe cases to reduce treatment time. *Disadvantages* • Takes 6–24 mo. • Retention may be a problem depending on severity of bite problem and habits. • Usually requires wearing a retainer indefinitely.	*Advantages* • May create the illusion of straightness • Can sometimes minimally reduce protrusion • Completed in 1 office visit *Disadvantages* • Does not correct the problem

BONDING	PORCELAIN VENEERS	CROWNS
Advantages • Improves color and shape of teeth • Completed in 1 office visit *Disadvantages* • Does not correct bite problem • Can chip or stain • May need replacement every 3–8 years	*Advantages* • Improve color and shape of teeth *Disadvantages* • Do not correct bite problem • Can chip or fracture • May need replacement every 5–12 years	*Advantages* • Can be good option to correct closed bite. • In certain cases, crowning back teeth can improve bite and facial esthetics by creating space for more natural anterior teeth. *Disadvantages* • May be difficult to open bite. • Require tooth reduction • May need replacement every 5–15 years. • Require a local anesthetic.
Advantages • Can sometimes build out upper teeth to widen arch • Completed in 1 office visit *Disadvantages* • Can chip or stain • May need replacement every 3–8 years • Does not correct defective bite • Only indicated for mild conditions	*Advantages* • Can sometimes build out upper teeth to widen arch *Disadvantages* • Can fracture more easily in severe crossbites	*Advantages* • Can alter shape and color of teeth. • In rare cases, crowning both upper and lower teeth can improve or even correct some crossbites. *Disadvantages* • Require a local anesthetic. • Require tooth reduction. • Do not correct the defect. • May need replacement every 5–15 years.
Advantages • Can lengthen the upper teeth in mild conditions • Improves color and shape of teeth • Completed in 1 office visit *Disadvantages* • Limited amount of benefit • Does not improve lip position • Can chip or stain • May need replacement every 3–8 years	*Advantages* • Can lengthen the teeth in mild conditions • Improve color and shape of teeth *Disadvantages* • Limited amount of benefit • Does not improve lip position • Can chip or fracture • May need replacement every 5–12 years	*Advantages* • Can lengthen the teeth in mild conditions • Improve color and shape of teeth *Disadvantages* • Limited amount of benefit • Require tooth reduction • May need replacement every 5–15 years • Require a local anesthetic
Advantages • Completed in 1 office visit. • May slightly improve alignment. *Disadvantages* • Teeth may appear and feel thicker. • Can chip or stain. • May need replacement every 3–8 years.	*Advantages* • May slightly improve alignment. *Disadvantages* • Teeth may appear and feel thicker. • Can chip or fracture. • May need replacement every 5–12 years.	*Advantages* • Can improve the angle of teeth as well as color and shape *Disadvantages* • Cannot compensate for differences in upper and lower jawbones • May need replacement every 5–15 years • Require tooth reduction • May involve removal of nerves in teeth • Require a local anesthetic

Solution 1 Orthodontics

NEED TO MAKE A MOVE?

Orthodontics repositions the teeth so that they come together properly, and it is by far the best treatment for most bite problems. Orthodontics is the longest-lasting and most conservative treatment option; however, it does require a significant time commitment. In some cases, orthognathic surgery is combined with orthodontics to achieve faster and better-looking results.

> How It's Done
  see page 231

Your teeth, only better » This television personality wanted to enhance his smile. With orthodontic expansion of his arch and repositioning of his teeth, a good-looking smile that harmonized with the rest of his face was achieved.

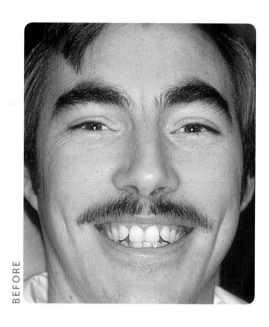

BEFORE

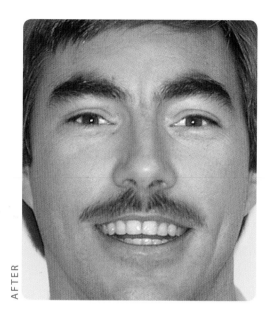

AFTER

expert tip Play it safe!

Whether it is accomplished using traditional brackets or clear matrices (such as Invisalign), orthodontics remains one of the most economical dental treatments. In addition, it is an important first step that will help your cosmetic dentist achieve the best possible esthetic and functional result, no matter what the next stage of treatment involves—bonding, veneers, or all-ceramic crowns.

8

Beauty from every angle » This 13-year-old girl found it difficult to close her mouth because of her protruding teeth. Two years of orthodontic treatment resulted in not only straighter teeth but also a much improved facial profile.

BEFORE

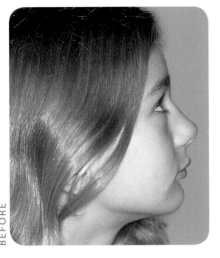
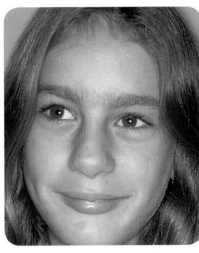
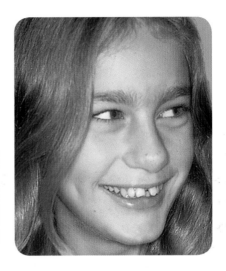

AFTER

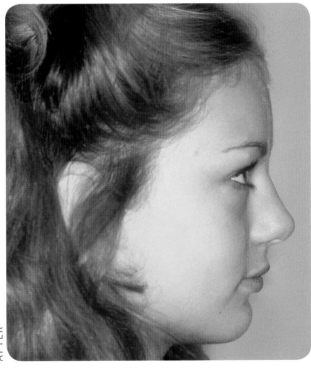
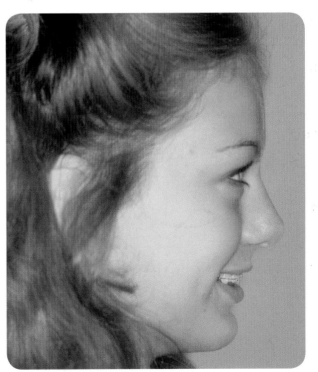

Solution 2 Cosmetic Contouring

LOOKING FOR A FINISHING TOUCH?

Cosmetic contouring, or reshaping the natural teeth to create an illusion of straightness, can sometimes be the easiest way to correct problems associated with poor bites, particularly in cases of minor crowding or uneven tooth lengths. However, cosmetic contouring by itself cannot solve most bite problems; it is usually at best a compromise solution or a final touch to improve the shapes of teeth following other treatment.

Even out your smile » This 31-year-old state beauty contestant winner had extremely long canines. After a 1-hour cosmetic contouring appointment in which the canines were reshaped, the patient's smile line was improved.

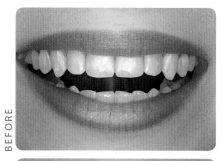

BEFORE

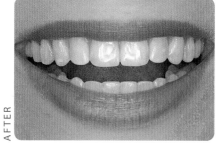

AFTER

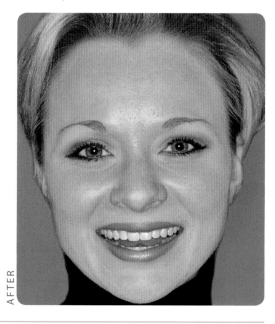

AFTER

A slight change can make a big difference » This dental hygienist's large overlapping front teeth accentuated her protruded upper jaw. Although orthodontics would have been the ideal solution, the patient opted for cosmetic contouring of the two front teeth, which helped give the illusion that the teeth were more in line and also much thinner, helping to reduce the appearance of protrusion.

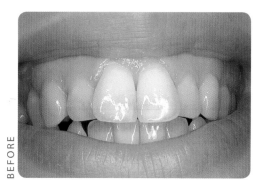

BEFORE

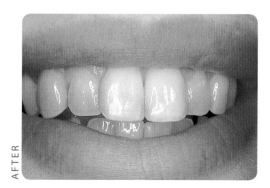

AFTER

8

Solution 3 Bonding

A winning smile » A bad bite can contribute to an asymmetrical smile line. This beauty contestant wanted to improve her smile for an upcoming pageant. Composite resin bonding and cosmetic contouring were performed. The final result shows just how much a new smile can contribute to total facial harmony and success in life. (She won the pageant a few days later.)

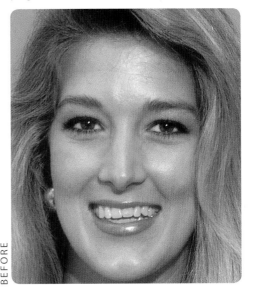

BEFORE

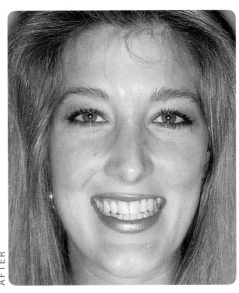

AFTER

Fill out your smile » A sunken-in look spoiled the smile of this otherwise handsome 45-year-old businessman. The inward angle of the teeth made them look shorter than they really were, and he didn't like the shiny silver filling on the right side. Composite resin bonding was used on the ten upper teeth, creating a new smile in just one appointment.

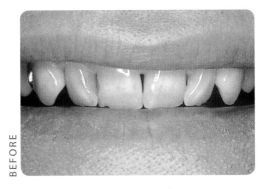

BEFORE

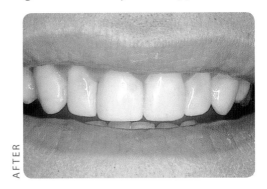

AFTER

CAN BONDING IMPROVE YOUR BITE?

Bonding, combined with cosmetic contouring, can be used for certain types of crossbites to build out the upper teeth and reshape the lower teeth so that they're in an improved relationship. Or, in select cases, bonding can be used to build out lower front teeth, which can help diminish the look of protruding upper teeth. However, bonding is generally a weak compromise treatment for most bite problems. It's more effective as a way to make discolored, chipped, crowded, worn, or irregularly spaced teeth look better in the existing bite relationship.

> How It's Done
> *see page 217*

Solution 4 Porcelain Veneers

LOOKING FOR A **FULLER** SMILE?

Porcelain veneers offer a good compromise solution for a narrow arch. If the teeth are in good health, they can easily be built out, which accomplishes the goal of a wider smile. Using a brighter shade of porcelain can also help to give the illusion of a fuller smile. However, if the teeth have many defective restorations, crowns may be a better option.

▷ How It's Done
see pages 218–219

An attractive smile speaks for itself » This minister wanted to improve his speaking appearance, which was marred by a crooked smile. The smile line was greatly improved by first reshaping the existing teeth and then placing ten porcelain veneers. The new smile resulted in an overall more handsome look.

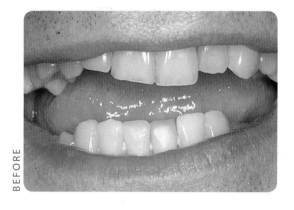
BEFORE

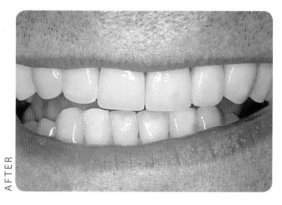
AFTER

Grinding can ruin a good smile » This man was uncomfortable with the spaces between his teeth. In addition, his grinding habit had made the teeth too short and irregular. He wanted his teeth to look better, but natural—not too white. Since the patient also wanted to preserve his natural teeth as much as possible, very thin veneers with a slightly brighter shade were chosen. The result pleased the patient, who now gets compliments on his smile.

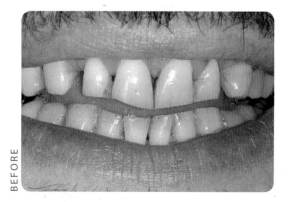
BEFORE

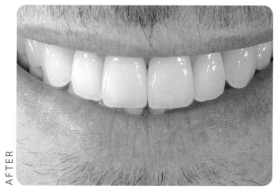
AFTER

8

A brighter, fuller smile » This actress and model was displeased with the dark spaces (she called them "caves") that she saw on each side of her mouth when she smiled. The solution to this cosmetic problem involved building out both the front and back teeth with lighter-colored porcelain veneers. Lighter-colored teeth appear to stand out, whereas darkly stained teeth appear to recede.

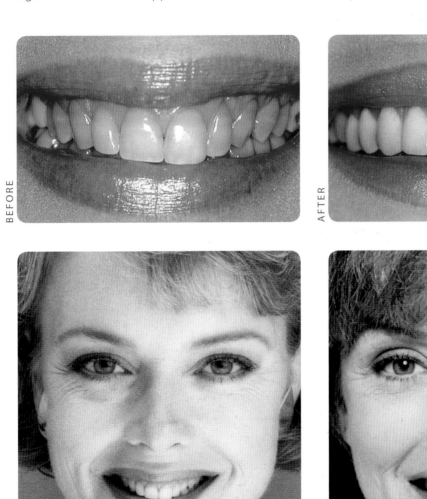

BEFORE

AFTER

BEFORE

AFTER

Solution 5 Crowns

CAN CROWNS BRING BACK YOUR BITE?

In cases of extreme wear due to age or bruxism, crowns rather than orthodontics may be the treatment of choice. Crowns can also be used in combination with orthodontics to move the lower teeth back or improve the look of protruding upper teeth.

Has your smile gone flat? » This 61-year-old executive's front and back teeth had been worn to the point of being almost flat and too small for his face. All the teeth were crowned to restore the lost tooth structure and help create a younger-looking and more handsome smile.

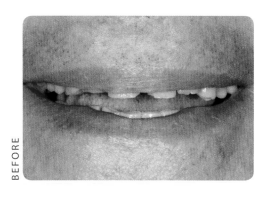

BEFORE

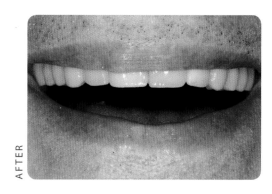

AFTER

Don't let your smile age you » This 25-year-old male model had an older-appearing ("reverse") smile line because his canines were longer than his other front teeth. The upper four front teeth were crowned. Notice how making the two front teeth longer helps create a more youthful and appealing smile line.

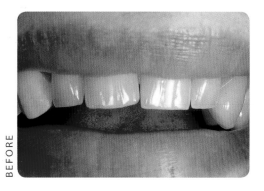

BEFORE

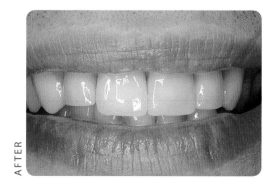

AFTER

WHY LENGTHEN YOUR UPPER TEETH?

These diagrams illustrate how the upper teeth can be lengthened (using bonding, porcelain veneers, or crowns) to provide a more attractive smile line.

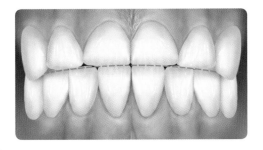 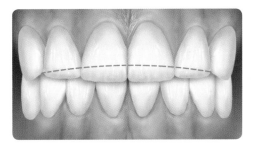 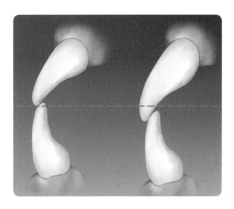

A combination approach to longer, prettier teeth » This 57-year-old woman had worn her back teeth down so much that the front teeth also began to wear. As a first step, a removable appliance was created to help determine if the bite could be slightly opened to permit longer front teeth and to allow the jaw muscles to relax and be more comfortable. After approximately 3 months, the teeth were ready to be rebuilt in a new relationship. All the back teeth were restored with porcelain-fused-to-metal crowns. The front teeth were bonded with composite resin, which produced a prettier new color and shape along with more tooth length. The combined approach greatly improved her smile as well as her overall appearance.

BEFORE

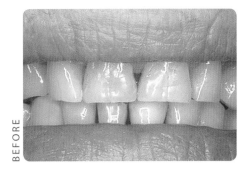

AFTER

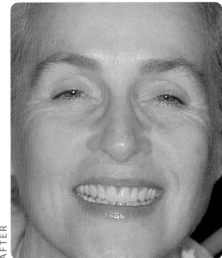

WHICH SOLUTION IS BEST FOR **YOU?**

	ORTHODONTICS	COSMETIC CONTOURING
TREATMENT TIME	6–24 mo in most cases	1 hour
MAINTENANCE	• Brush and floss daily with special care. • Have checkups 2–4 times per year after movement is completed. • Wear retainer indefinitely at least a few nights per week.	• Brush and floss daily. • Have a professional cleaning 2–4 times per year.
RESULTS	Bite problems can usually be solved by realigning the teeth so they meet properly.	Can improve minor bite problems within a matter of minutes and can sometimes prevent headaches or other problems associated with bad bites
TREATMENT LONGEVITY*	Generally permanent if retainer is worn at least a few nights per week	Indefinite
COST†	$1,500 to $7,500	$250 to $2,500 per arch
ADVANTAGES	• Permanent results for most people if retainer is worn • Can help cure or prevent TMJ pain • Improves ability to bite • Can improve lip position	• Good for esthetically shaping the teeth as a final touch. • Completed in 1 office visit. • Can reshape teeth in opposite arch to help improve bite. • Teeth may appear straighter.
DISADVANTAGES	• Time consuming. • Usually requires wearing a retainer indefinitely. • May need to be combined with orthognathic surgery to be fully effective. • Retention may be a problem depending on severity of bite problem and habits.	• Does not correct the bite problem

*This estimate is based on the author's clinical experience combined with three university research studies and insurance company estimates. Your own experience could be different, depending on many factors, only some of which you and your dentist can control.

†Fees will vary from dentist to dentist based on the difficulty of the procedure, patient problems, patient dental and medical history, expectations, and dentist qualifications, including technical and artistic expertise.

‡Expect to pay extra for esthetic temporaries.

8

BONDING	PORCELAIN VENEERS	CROWNS
About 1 hour or less per tooth	2 office visits; 4–6 hours each for most cases of up to10 teeth	Usually 2 office visits; 1–4 hours each for up to 4 teeth (more time for additional teeth or more extensive treatment)
• Have a professional cleaning 2–4 times per year depending on amount of stain. • Brush and floss daily. • Bite carefully to avoid torque.	• Have a professional cleaning 2–4 times per year depending on amount of stain. • Brush and floss daily. • Bite carefully to avoid torque.	• Brush and floss daily. • Have a professional cleaning 2–4 times per year. • Avoid biting down on hard foods and ice. • Get yearly fluoride treatments or more if necessary.
A good quick compromise in certain cases	Depending on the severity of the problem, may create a more esthetic smile even if the actual bite problem is not corrected	Correct misaligned teeth that are causing a bad bite, sometimes within a matter of weeks
5–8 years (directly related to fractures, problems with tissues, decay, and patient home care)	5–12 years (directly related to fractures, problems with tissues, decay, and patient home care)	5–15 years (directly related to fractures, tissue problems, decay, and patient home care)
$500 to $1,750 per tooth	$950 to $3,500 per tooth[‡]	$950 to $3,500 per tooth[‡]
• Can improve color and shape of teeth • Completed in 1 office visit • Can sometimes build out upper teeth to give the appearance of a wider arch • Can lengthen the teeth • May slightly improve alignment • Less costly than porcelain veneers or crowns	• Can improve color and shape of teeth • Completed in 1 office visit • Can sometimes build out upper teeth to give the appearance of a wider arch • Can lengthen the teeth • May slightly improve alignment • Less tooth reduction required than crowning	• Can improve angle, shape, and color of teeth. • Crowning back teeth can reshape bite and improve facial esthetics. • Can lengthen the teeth.
• Does not correct the bite problem. • Can chip or stain. • May need replacement every 3–8 years. • Only indicated for mild conditions. • Teeth may appear and feel thicker.	• Does not correct the bite problem. • Can chip or fracture. • May need replacement every 5–12 years. • Only indicated for mild conditions. • Teeth may appear and feel thicker. • More expensive than bonding.	• Tooth form is altered (most of the tooth enamel is removed). • May need replacement in 5–15 years. • Requires a local anesthetic. • May not correct the bite problem. • May involve removal of nerves in teeth to accomplish better tooth position and improved lip line. • More expensive than bonding or veneers.

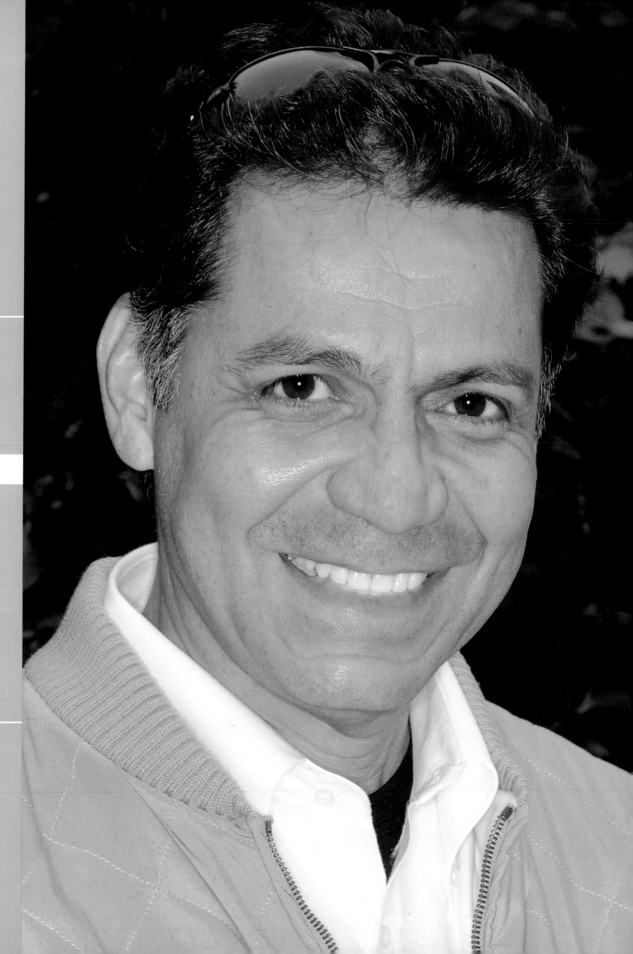

9

It's About Time

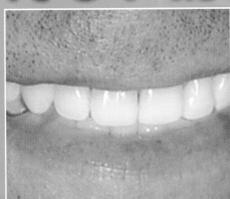

You can look years younger with cosmetic dentistry!

Consumers spend billions of dollars each year on services and products designed to make them look more attractive. Countless women—and increasing numbers of men—have facelifts and other surgical procedures in an effort to enhance their appearance and remain competitive in job markets where looking youthful is an asset. While many patients benefit from plastic surgery, others could be helped with cosmetic dentistry alone. After all, your smile is one of the most important parts of your face. If your smile is attractive and healthy looking, it will take years off your appearance. If, on the other hand, your smile reveals worn, discolored, chipped, or missing teeth, you'll look older than you should, and no amount of plastic surgery can change that.

If you'd like to take years off your smile—and your overall looks—ask your dentist about cosmetic procedures that can help. Your chronological age should never stand between you and a more pleasing appearance.

HOW CAN YOU LOOK AND FEEL YOUNGER?

Dentistry's role in improving appearance is often misunderstood and underrated. For example, many people believe that only dentures can alter the appearance of their smile, yet nothing could be further from the truth. Such cost-effective techniques as cosmetic contouring, bleaching, or bonding often work wonders—typically in a single office visit!

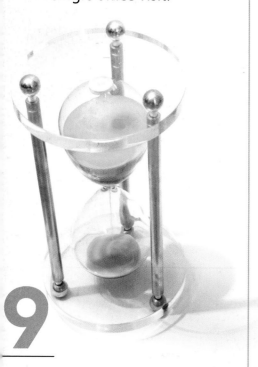

10 Tips to Keep Your Smile Young

1. Watch for unnatural wear and avoid grinding your teeth.
2. Take preventive oral hygiene seriously to avoid gum and bone loss.
3. Replace faulty fillings before they cause problems.
4. If crowns or bridges are worn down, replace them.
5. Lighten any discolored teeth.
6. Replace any missing teeth as soon as possible.
7. Correct a bad bite.
8. Never chew ice or hard candy or suck on lemons.
9. Ask your dentist for a video intraoral exam.
10. Avoid abrasive habits such as aggressive toothbrushing.

smile 101 What makes a smile look old?

As we age, the edges of the front teeth wear until these teeth are about the same length as the others. At the same time, the upper and lower lips lose muscle tone. The upper lip may sag, covering more or all of the upper teeth. The lower lip may also drop, allowing more of the lower teeth to show. The teeth become darker in color. These conditions create an older-looking smile.

expert tip It all starts with the smile!

The best way to obtain a more youthful look is by combining the advantages of cosmetic dentistry, cosmetology, and plastic surgery—in that order. First, improve your smile. Next, try following the expert beauty and hairstyle tips in chapter 12 to update your look. If you still have concerns, such as wrinkles or sagging skin, explore your options in plastic surgery with a qualified plastic surgeon (see chapter 11).

Never stop caring!

As they get older, some people stop taking proper care of themselves, including their teeth. If this sounds like you, remember that it's never too late to start taking care of yourself again. Many older adults today are seeking treatment to correct dental problems and improve their appearance. If you have friends or family members who no longer take an interest in their looks, share this book with them. Let them know how much better they can feel with an updated smile. You could be a tremendous help in improving not only their appearance but also their outlook on life.

WHAT YOU SHOULD KNOW

PREVENTION: THE BEST WAY TO FIGHT THE YEARS

You can keep your smile intact for a lifetime. Good oral hygiene—including toothbrushing, flossing, and regular visits to the dentist—will help keep teeth, gums, and bone in good health. Here are some tips on how to keep your teeth healthy:

▶ If you're not sure that you're brushing correctly, ask your dentist or hygienist to show you how. Although some loss of tooth structure due to mechanical wear is inevitable, incorrect toothbrushing often accelerates this process.

▶ Purchase chewable disclosing tablets that allow you to see the plaque you missed when brushing by revealing those areas in red.

▶ With the advice of your dentist, consider purchasing a site-specific rotary cleaning device. Research has shown that many people can improve their tooth-cleaning effectiveness with an electric toothbrush.

▶ Choose a dentist who offers an aggressive program of preventive maintenance. This should include three or four professional tooth cleanings per year, proper home care, monitoring of plaque control, periodontal probing, and referral to specialists such as periodontists when needed.

Cosmetic Contouring

WHY SPEND A FORTUNE?

The most economical way to correct teeth that are simply worn down is with cosmetic contouring. The upper teeth are reshaped to give the appearance that they are longer than they really are.

smile 101 What causes tooth wear?

Often teeth wear more quickly than they should due to factors other than aging. Some people have incorrect bites or a habit of grinding their teeth, either of which can contribute to a wearing down of tooth structure. If your teeth are worn down, there are several ways to correct the problem. You can lengthen the upper incisors with bonding or porcelain veneers and shorten the lower incisors. Alternatively, the upper teeth can be contoured to give an illusion that the front two teeth are longer than they actually are. You can also be fitted with a bite appliance if you grind your teeth at night.

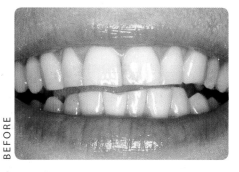

BEFORE

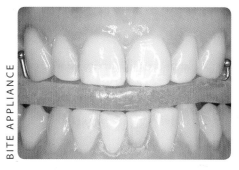

BITE APPLIANCE

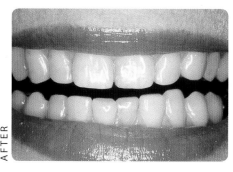

AFTER

Don't let worn teeth age you! » Bruxism, or grinding the teeth, was the chief cause of wear for this 31-year-old executive. In addition to poor dental esthetics, she suffered constant headaches as well as neck and back discomfort. The diagnosis was a temporomandibular joint disorder (TMD). A removable appliance was made to correct the TMD and prevent further tooth wear. Following 3 months of treatment to alleviate the TMD symptoms and relax the muscles, the square, masculine-looking upper and lower teeth were cosmetically contoured to produce a prettier, more feminine smile.

9

Solution 2 Bonding

Eliminate staining and asymmetry for a younger look » This woman realized that her stained and uneven teeth were aging her smile. Following composite resin bonding and cosmetic contouring of the upper and lower teeth, her teeth look lighter and more even, and her smile is more youthful.

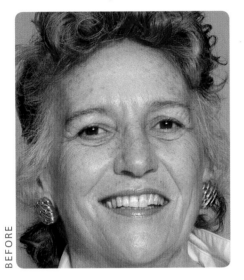

BEFORE

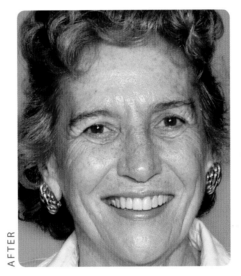

AFTER

GET A YOUNGER SMILE IN HOURS!

Bonding the front surfaces of worn teeth gives the smile a more youthful and healthy appearance in a matter of hours. Although bonding eventually must be redone, the procedure is less expensive than porcelain veneers or crowns.

> ▸ How It's Done
> *see page 217*

Keep it natural » This woman's worn and discolored teeth had faulty fillings that spoiled an otherwise attractive smile. However, she did not want to have crowns on her "good" teeth if at all possible. Her six upper front teeth were lengthened with composite resin bonding. It would have been a mistake to lighten her teeth too much, since it would have made them look unnatural. The bonding required only polishing every 6 to 12 months for 9 years before replacement was necessary.

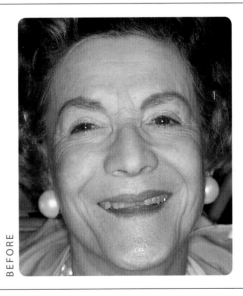

BEFORE

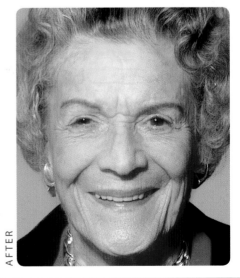

AFTER

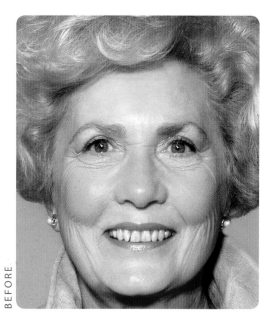

BEFORE

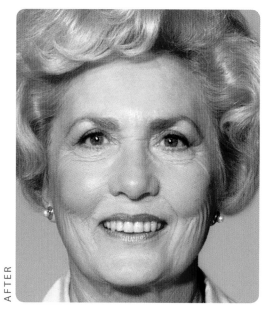

AFTER

Soften your smile » This woman was displeased about her discolored and twisted teeth. In addition, she felt that the sharp points of her teeth made them look like fangs. Her six front teeth were first contoured and then bonded to make them appear straighter. Notice how a softer look was achieved just by contouring the bonded teeth.

Looking younger on a schedule » This man became acutely aware that his discolored, worn, and spaced teeth were making him look older than his years and wanted it corrected as quickly as possible for a special event. Direct composite resin bonding was chosen as an interim solution because it could be completed without tooth reduction in a single office visit. Although treatment was focused on the upper teeth, the lower spaces were closed as well, which made the patient even more pleased with his new younger look. Seven months later the bonding was replaced with porcelain veneers and all-ceramic crowns for greater strength and longevity.

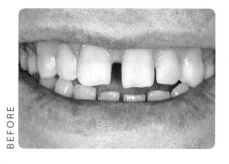

BEFORE

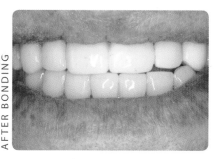

AFTER BONDING

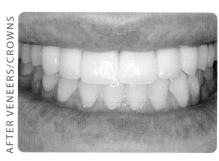

AFTER VENEERS/CROWNS

9

Solution 3 Porcelain Veneers

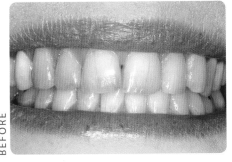

BEFORE

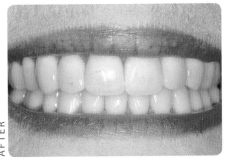

AFTER

Dark teeth can age you » This 58-year-old woman felt much younger than her age. However, her darkly stained teeth made her appear much older. Porcelain veneers in a much brighter shade combined with posterior all-ceramic crowns gave her a smile that went with her pretty face.

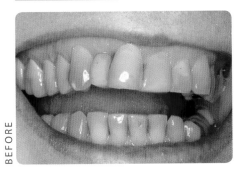

BEFORE

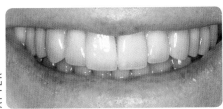

AFTER

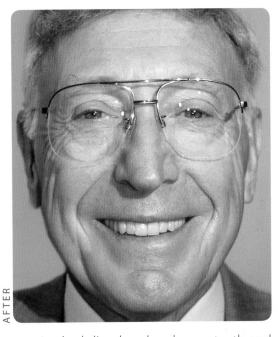

AFTER

The power of a good smile » This executive had discolored and worn teeth and irregular-looking gum tissue, resulting in an aged smile. After the gums were cosmetically and functionally improved, five porcelain veneers were placed, along with posterior crowns and inlays. The result was lighter teeth and improved tooth shape and arch alignment. Most importantly, the patient looked as young as he felt.

GET THE TEETH YOU ALWAYS WANTED!

Discolored and worn front teeth are two of the telltale signs of aging. If the teeth are otherwise in relatively good health, porcelain veneers can be an excellent treatment for providing a younger look. Your bite may be the deciding factor if veneers or ceramic crowns are the best solution. Many times cosmetic contouring of the lower teeth can be combined with longer porcelain veneers on the upper teeth to bring back that youthful appearance.

> ⊳ | How It's Done
> *see pages 218–219*

Solution 4 **Crowns**

For patients with extensive tooth wear—regardless of the cause—maximum improvement is usually obtained with crowns. It may even be possible to restore your bite to its previous condition. In addition, all-ceramic crowns are made from a beautiful material that can completely mask staining and can straighten and replace worn teeth simultaneously.

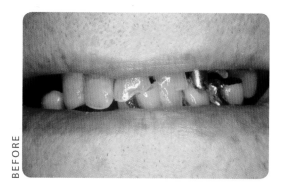

> How It's Done
> *see pages 220–225*

what to eXpect

REBUILDING YOUR BITE

- If your bite has collapsed, the first step may involve wearing an acrylic or composite resin bite appliance. If you can tolerate this appliance, the chances are excellent that you will be able to rebuild your bite with crowns or bridges.

- The second step is to wear plastic temporary crowns or bridges to replace the bite appliance. (Note that some dentists choose to proceed directly to this step without the use of an appliance.)

- The last step involves replacing these temporary restorations with the final—and more durable—crowns or bridges.

A good smile brings great comfort » Although this 69-year-old retired executive was in poor health, he wanted to improve the function of his teeth as well as his appearance. For patients who are ailing, a compromise treatment plan can improve their smile with a minimal investment of time and money. Temporary crowns and bridges on all the existing teeth were made in a lighter color to rebuild his teeth and improve his appearance. The patient was immediately satisfied with his good-looking smile.

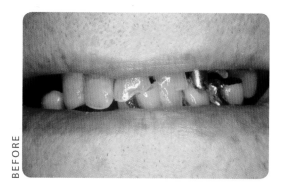

BEFORE

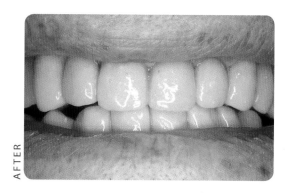

AFTER

9

expert tip Don't extract healthy teeth!

Never have your teeth extracted if there is sufficient bone to save them, even if only a root remains. However, if your bone is diseased, you may need periodontal surgery to save your teeth. Surgery is often worthwhile, since good tooth roots usually function better than implants.

When your smile looks good, so do you! » This businessman had worn his front crowns so much that the gold beneath the acrylic veneer on the right lateral incisor showed. The other acrylic veneer crowns were discolored, making him look older than he was. New porcelain crowns with a lighter and more youthful look produced an attractive smile.

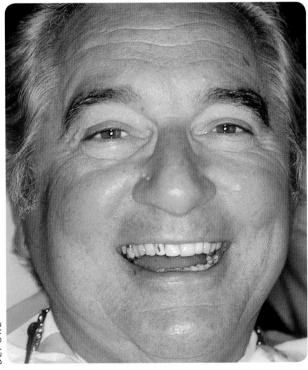

BEFORE

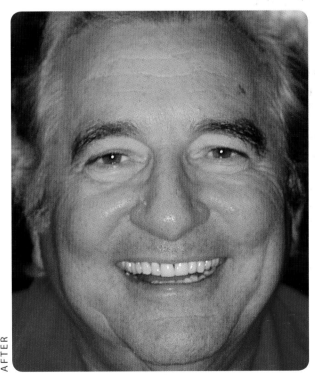

AFTER

Solution 5 **Orthodontics**

TIME TO MAKE YOUR MOVE?

According to the American Association of Orthodontists, more than one in every five orthodontic patients is an adult. The availability of clear ceramic brackets and plastic matrices makes orthodontics a more acceptable alternative than in years past. If it takes tooth repositioning with orthodontics to improve your smile, do it if you can. You're never too old for tooth movement. Your bite will improve and so will your appearance.

> How It's Done
> *see page 231*

see page 231

9

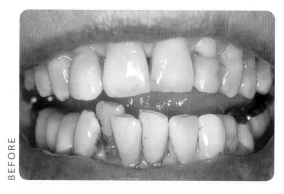

BEFORE

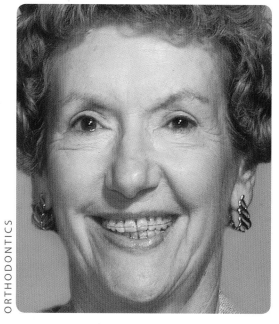

ORTHODONTICS

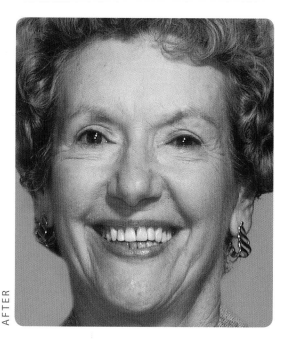

AFTER

It's never too late » This 65-year-old woman's crowded and discolored teeth made her look older than she felt. Ten months of orthodontic treatment helped reposition her front teeth, then bonding with composite resin lightened the teeth and helped mask the stained fillings. No one is too old to have teeth repositioned.

A younger smile to last a lifetime » This 56-year-old health-conscious woman wanted to properly correct her bad bite. She opted for orthodontics with tooth-colored brackets, and her teeth were repositioned in 18 months. Composite resin bonding was then done to improve her smile. Twenty-four years after orthodontic treatment, her smile still looks great. Although the bonding required special care and maintenance to achieve such longevity, the tooth repositioning was essentially a permanent solution.

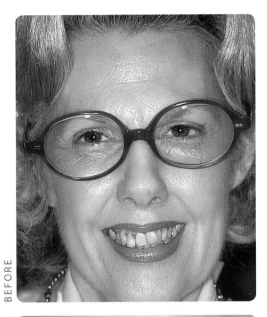

BEFORE

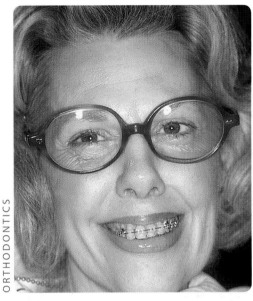

ORTHODONTICS

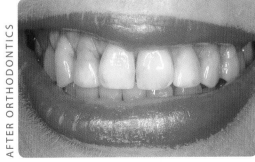

AFTER ORTHODONTICS

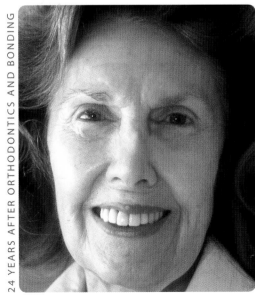

24 YEARS AFTER ORTHODONTICS AND BONDING

Solution 6 **Dentures**

IS TOOTH LOSS AGING YOUR SMILE?

If some or all of your teeth have been lost or can't be restored and need to be extracted, it's important that you not allow too much time to lag between tooth loss and tooth replacement. Tooth loss causes the face to collapse and the mouth to sink in. At the same time, the nose appears to drop down toward the chin. Deep lines begin to form in the creases of this collapsed skin, adding years to the face. Dentures can help you avoid all of these problems and give you a brand new smile.

 expert tip Dentures don't last forever!

Because dentures fracture and chip much more easily than do natural teeth, you may want to have a spare set, particularly if you travel a lot. It's worth the extra cost to have teeth when you need a repair. Although it can be expensive, you may want to get an exact duplicate of the original denture if you require a perfect smile at all times. Also remember that if the teeth are made of acrylic—and most of them are—they may show wear within 3 to 6 years. If you grind your teeth, you can expect to show tooth wear in half that time. Be sure to have your dentures rebased, relined, or remade when they show signs of wear so that your smile remains attractive and functional.

Is your old denture wearing on you? » Wear on the upper denture combined with lack of proper lip support made this woman look older than her 48 years. A new full upper denture provided increased lip support and created a more youthful smile line.

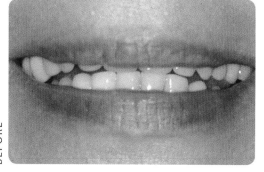

BEFORE

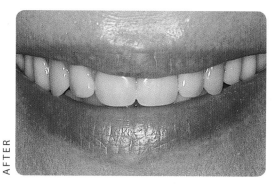

AFTER

9

WHAT YOU SHOULD KNOW

WHAT TYPE OF DENTURE DO YOU NEED?

Immediate denture

Immediate dentures are measured for size with the natural teeth intact, and they are placed the same day as your remaining teeth are extracted. With this type of denture, you skip the try-in stages that accompany the fitting of other models. Because gums and bone tend to shrink after extraction, these dentures may become loose. However, an additional inner lining can be placed inside the dentures to make them fit. This means the replacement time for immediate dentures is often shorter than that for conventional models. It may also mean additional charges for adjustments and lining.

Conventional denture

Fitting conventional dentures typically requires three to six office visits after all of the teeth have been removed and the tissue has healed. During these visits, you will be able to evaluate the fit and look of the dentures. Your dentist will advise you on color, tooth type, and lip position. Keep in mind that if the color is too white, the dentures will look artificial. Conventional dentures cost about the same as immediate dentures. Some dentists also include the cost of later adjustments in their fee.

Custom denture

Custom-made dentures have specially shaded teeth and gums and other characteristics, even gold or silver fillings, that duplicate the original teeth. Because of this, they are the most esthetic, but also the most expensive, type of denture.

Solution 7 Implants

If you've lost teeth due to trauma or periodontal disease, it may still be possible to replace them with dental implants. There are so many advantages to replacing one or all of your missing teeth with dental implants that this treatment has become the therapy of choice. Even if you've lost supporting bone, many times it's possible to use a bone graft to restore the bone and then place the implants later.

▶— How It's Done
see pages 228–230

Nothing to fear » A self-described dental phobic, this grandmother had let her teeth become discolored and loose. A caring professional team plus oral conscious sedation helped her overcome her fear of treatment during a 6-hour implant surgery. She left surgery with an attractive removable bridge supported by six implants. The new self-confident attitude she gained from knowing how great she looked made the experience worthwhile.

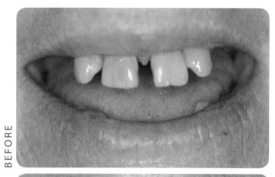

BEFORE

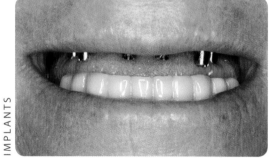

IMPLANTS

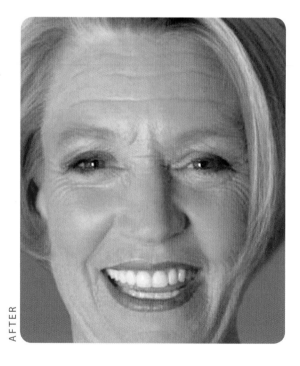

AFTER

9

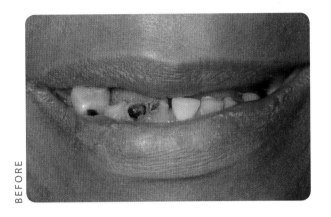

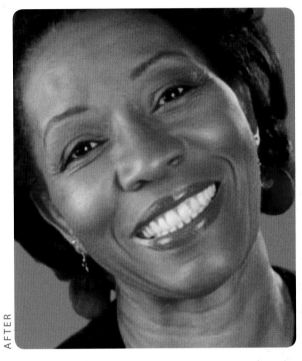

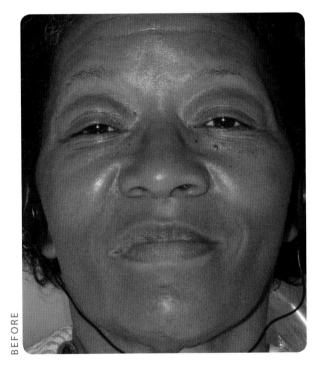

A neglected smile can lead to low self-esteem » This 61-year-old artist was so embarrassed by her teeth that she would usually cover her smile with her hand. Since the teeth were beyond repair, implant-retained dentures were selected as the treatment of choice. The hopeless teeth were extracted, then bone was surgically added to improve the fit of new dentures. A more youthful and healthier-looking smile was designed with four implants in the lower arch, along with a removable upper denture. Now her friends tell her how amazing she looks, and her paintings have been rejuvenated as well!

WHICH SOLUTION IS BEST FOR **YOU?**

COSMETIC CONTOURING	BONDING	VENEERS OR CROWNS
TREATMENT TIME		
About 1 hour	About 1 hour per tooth	*Veneers:* 2 office visits; about 4 hours each *Crowns:* 2–3 office visits; about 1–2 hours each per tooth
MAINTENANCE		
Brush and floss daily.	• Have a professional cleaning 3–4 times per year. • Eat wisely—bonded teeth can chip easily. • Push floss in and pull it through teeth rather than popping it out. • See dentist for repair as necessary.	• Have a professional cleaning 3–4 times per year. • Avoid biting down on hard foods and ice. • Brush and floss daily. • Get yearly fluoride treatments.
RESULTS		
Can create a more youthful smile in certain patients	Can lengthen front teeth to create a younger smile line and can repair distracting chips and discoloration	*Veneers:* Can lengthen front teeth to create a younger smile line *Crowns:* May be the best way to produce a more youthful smile
TREATMENT LONGEVITY*		
Indefinite	5–8 years	5–15 years
COST†		
$350 to $2,500 per arch	$250 to $2,500 per tooth	$950 to $3,500 per tooth‡
ADVANTAGES		
• Quickest option for certain patients, especially those with worn teeth • Least expensive option • Permanent results	• Can lengthen and lighten teeth at the same time to create a younger-looking smile	*Veneers:* • Can lengthen and lighten teeth at the same time • Long lasting • Require less maintenance than bonding *Crowns:* • Can be the best solution, especially for creating good proportions in the smile • Good restorative method if bite needs opening
DISADVANTAGES		
• May not correct the problem • Usually a compromise rather than an ideal option	• May not correct the problem • Usually a compromise rather than an ideal option • Must be repaired and maintained • Requires more caution when biting	*Veneers:* • May not correct the problem • Usually a compromise rather than an ideal option *Crowns:* • Require tooth reduction • More expensive than contouring or bonding

9

156

*This estimate is based on the author's clinical experience combined with three university research studies and insurance company estimates. Your own experience could be different, depending on many factors, only some of which you and your dentist can control.

†Fees will vary from dentist to dentist based on the difficulty of the procedure, patient problems, patient dental and medical history, expectations, and dentist qualifications, including technical and artistic expertise.

‡Expect to pay extra for esthetic temporaries.

ORTHODONTICS	DENTURES	IMPLANTS
6 mo to 3 years	2–5 office visits	*Two-stage implant:* 1 visit for surgery, 3 mo later implant uncovered, then crown made *Immediate implant:* 1 visit for surgery and temporary crown made, 3 mo later final crown made
• Brush and floss daily with special care. • Have checkups 2–4 times per year after movement is completed. • Wear retainer indefinitely at least a few nights per week.	• Have a checkup 2 times per year to monitor fit, tooth wear, and tissue. • Have dentures professionally cleaned.	• Have a prophylaxis appointment 4 times per year. • Follow a customized home care regimen. • Do not smoke.
Can be quite helpful in positioning the teeth to appear straighter and more youthful	Can easily make you appear much younger	Especially helpful for patients who have lost teeth, since it gives them the feeling of having their natural teeth back, but better.
Generally permanent if retainer is worn at least a few nights per week	Good initial results, but some wear will occur if teeth are acrylic	Indefinite
$3,500 to $9,000	• *Immediate:* $575 to $2,500 for upper and lower, plus surgical fees if required • *Custom-made:* $1,500 to $6,000 per arch	$2,000 to $7,000 with implant and crown
• Best method if there are jaw deformities, crowded teeth, large spaces, or bite problems	• If all teeth missing, quickest way to create a new, younger-looking smile	• Best way to restore missing teeth to create a natural- and younger-looking smile • Do not damage surrounding teeth • Preserve bone • Can outlast tooth- or tissue-supported bridges
• Usually requires wearing a retainer indefinitely	• On upper arch, denture acrylic covers entire palate. • Better to have implants if possible for greater chewing ability.	• Anterior implant may be a problem if there is severe bone loss. • May be contraindicated for smokers or slow-healing patients such as bisphosphonate users.

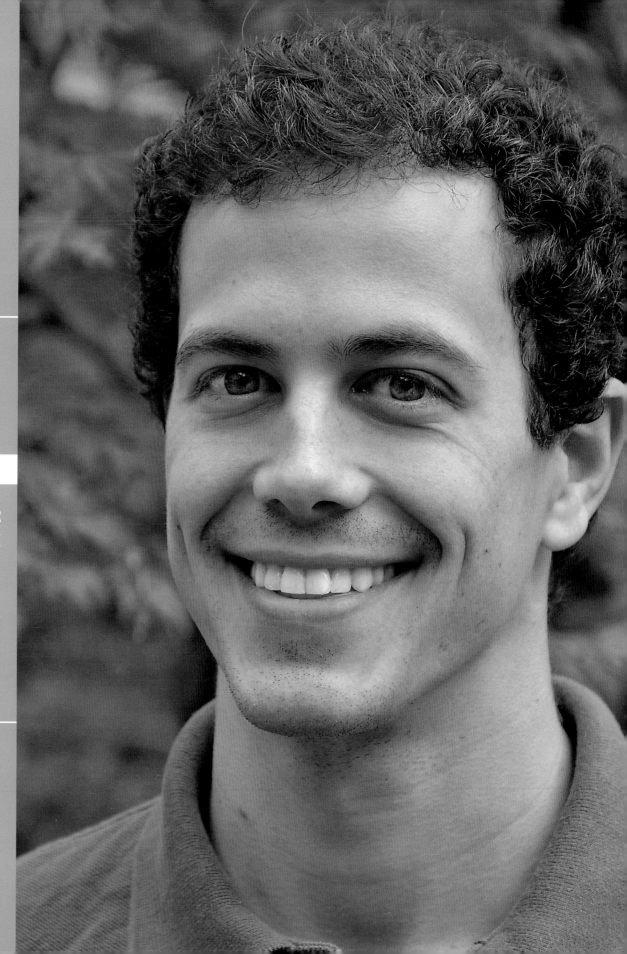

10

FIND OUT . . .

HOW THE HEALTH OF YOUR
GUMS AFFECTS YOUR SMILE

WHAT TO DO IF YOU HAVE
TOO LITTLE OR TOO MUCH
GUM TISSUE

WHY HAVING ENOUGH
BONE IS IMPORTANT

Gumming up the Works

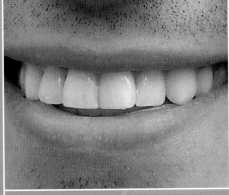

Are your gums keeping your smile from looking its best?

If you imagine your teeth as the canvas of a painting, then the gum tissue is the frame around the canvas. That means your gums can make or break your smile. You can have very attractive natural teeth, bonding, veneers, or crowns, but if your gum tissue is red, puffy, or bleeding, then the result is an unattractive smile. Also, if your gum tissue shrinks away from your beautiful restorations, leaving a black triangle where the gum used to be, you are left with an older-looking and unesthetic smile.

This chapter tells you everything you need to know to keep your gums healthy and what you can do if you have too much—or not enough—"pink" in your smile.

WHAT IS GUM DISEASE?

Gum disease, also called *periodontal disease*, is caused by excessive bacteria building up in the mouth. In the early stages, gums may bleed easily and appear red, tender, spongy, and slightly swollen. Eventually, the disease may lead to recession of the gums, destruction of the underlying bone, loosening of the teeth, and ultimately tooth loss. In addition, periodontal disease presents a major health risk. Research has shown that it has a strong connection with heart disease, lung disease, diabetes, and other systemic illnesses.

smile 101 — What are plaque and tartar?

The collection of bacteria and their by-products on the teeth is commonly referred to as plaque. If plaque is allowed to remain in the mouth for too long, the minerals from the saliva cause it to harden, forming what is known as *calculus* or *tartar*. The accumulation of either plaque or tartar can lead to gum disease. Therefore, it is important to remove any buildup on the teeth at regular intervals.

expert tip — Know your risk!

Certain systemic changes can increase your chances of getting gum disease. These include pregnancy, hormonal changes, psychological stress, and some drugs or medications.

GUM DISEASE is the primary cause of tooth loss in adults.

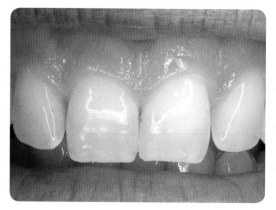

The picture of good health » Healthy gum tissue is usually pink, knife-edged, and stippled like an orange peel. Notice how it curves around the neck of the tooth and frames it. Various shades of pink may be characteristic of healthy tissue depending on a person's ethnic background and skin tone. Stippling may also vary according to age and sex.

what to eXpect

GUM DISEASE TREATMENT

- Plaque removal, accomplished through diligent home care (brushing, flossing, and other therapies prescribed by your dentist) and regular visits to your dentist or hygienist for professional cleanings, often prevents gum disease or stops it in its early stages.

- If gum disease is more advanced, professional root planing and curettage may be required. Root planing (also called *scaling*) is the removal of plaque and calculus from the tooth crowns and root surfaces. Curettage is the removal of the diseased gum tissue. These procedures, combined with meticulous home care, may be sufficient to control the disease, depending on its severity.

- In later stages of the disease, surgery is often required. The dentist surgically lifts sections of gum tissue, removes plaque and calculus, and corrects bone defects. The tissue is then positioned to allow more efficient cleaning. The procedure usually requires only a local anesthetic.

- If surgery reveals extreme bone loss, then bone grafting or guided bone regeneration (GBR) is sometimes required. These procedures are typically performed over the course of several appointments but in some cases may be done all at once with the use of conscious sedation or in a hospital or an outpatient facility with the aid of a general anesthetic.

Unhealthy gums can spoil a good smile » Treatment for this patient would consist of several office visits, usually with the hygienist. First, measurements would be taken to determine the extent of the disease. Then deep scaling, most likely with a local anesthetic, would be performed over a series of appointments. To maintain a healthy smile, she would need to brush and floss properly and consistently at home.

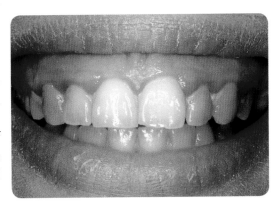

HOW IS GUM DISEASE TREATED?

Because it is difficult to cure advanced forms of gum disease, the sooner it is detected, the better. The objective of treatment is to stop its progression as quickly and effectively as possible. Therefore, if you have any of the symptoms mentioned, seek the help of your family dentist or a periodontist.

expert tip Prevention is best!

The best way to avoid gum disease is through careful home care. This includes regular brushing, flossing, rinsing, and gum massage. In other words, keep your mouth as clean as possible so that bacteria can't accumulate.

WHAT CAUSES
LOOSE TEETH?

Loose teeth don't always mean gum disease, but if when you press on your teeth they move back into your gums, gum disease is probably the culprit. If the disease has not progressed so far that the teeth are severely loose, then treatment of the inflamed and infected gums will usually correct the problem.

If your teeth are loose, your dentist may suggest splinting the teeth together with a bonding material so they can withstand the pressure of chewing while the gum and bone are healing. This is often an effective temporary solution that gives the teeth time to stabilize. If this is successful, interconnected crowns may eventually be placed on the loose teeth as well as those that adjoin them. This solution provides support while also allowing retention of most of the natural tooth structure.

Add strength and beauty to your smile » This 55-year-old woman had gum disease and underwent surgery to save her teeth. However, the teeth were still loose, and she was concerned about the resulting unattractive spaces between her teeth. Full crowns were made with extra porcelain to hide the spaces while also splinting the teeth together. The final result shows a new smile with whiter, more stabilized teeth and no spaces.

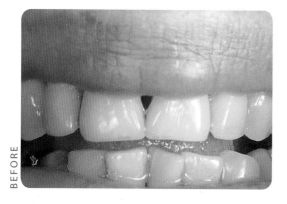

BEFORE

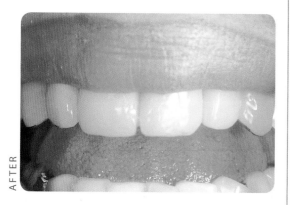

AFTER

10

Are you looking long in the tooth? » This woman had a high lip line that revealed the severely receding gum tissue on her right canine. Cosmetic gum surgery, which involved placement of a graft, was used to enhance both function and esthetics.

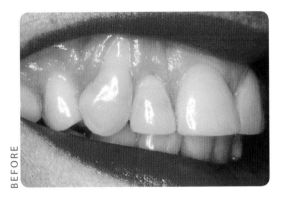

BEFORE

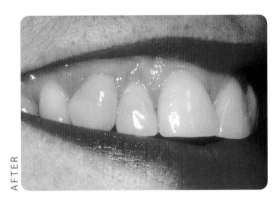

AFTER

 expert tip Hold on to your gums!

The best way to avoid tissue recession is to practice good oral hygiene at home and to have professional tooth cleanings three or four times each year. Also, begin proper cleaning immediately after a crown is placed even if the tissue is sore. If bacteria accumulate around the gum line, recession may occur.

WHAT CAUSES GUM LOSS?

Loss or recession of gum tissue can have a variety of causes, including gum disease, severe infection, trauma, or tooth extraction. When the gums shrink away from the teeth, the teeth appear longer, and unattractive spaces can show between them. Unfortunately, gum tissue doesn't usually grow back. Therefore, grafting of gum tissue is often performed either to correct the deformity or to prevent the recession from worsening.

WHAT YOU SHOULD KNOW

MASKING GUM LOSS

Full crowns, or sometimes porcelain veneers, can be used to mask a loss of interdental tissue but generally aren't recommended unless the teeth themselves need to be restored. Whenever possible, composite resin bonding is used to build up the teeth and fill in the spaces. Bonding is usually preferable to crowns because it's less costly and requires little tooth reduction. However, it must be repeated after several years and is susceptible to staining.

what to eXpect

RECEDING GUMS MAY EXPOSE CROWN MARGINS

If you have crowns and your gum tissue recedes, the previously hidden junction where tooth and crown meet may become visible (see page 224). The root of your tooth, which is typically darker than the crown, may be unsightly, or a metal or porcelain margin may show. Masking typically involves removing part of the crown and root and bonding over the area with composite resin to hide the metal margin or exposed root. However, because it's difficult to obtain a good esthetic match this way, a better alternative is to dull the metal slightly or hide it with a darker-colored composite resin. If the junction is porcelain and the root is dark, a better color match, although not a perfect one, will probably be obtained. However, the ideal solution is to replace the crown.

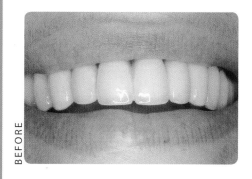

BEFORE

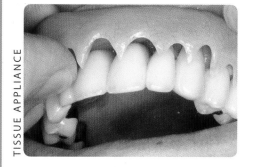

TISSUE APPLIANCE

Restore beauty with convenience » This 24-year-old student lost her four upper front teeth as well as supporting bone in a car accident. The teeth were replaced with a fixed bridge, but her high lip line revealed spaces between the teeth. A removable artificial tissue appliance was made. The pink acrylic, which closely matches her gum tissue, fits the shape of her teeth and locks into the spaces between them. It can be easily inserted or taken out and allows her to eat and speak normally.

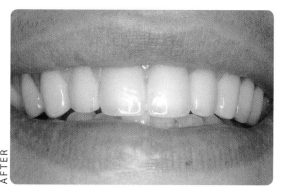

AFTER

Filling in the gaps » This 45-year-old television reporter wanted to hide the unsightly spaces between her teeth where gum tissue had been removed during periodontal surgery, but she did not want to have her teeth crowned. Her older fillings were removed, and composite resin bonding was placed around the necks of the front six teeth. In addition to concealing the spaces, the bonding material lightened her teeth.

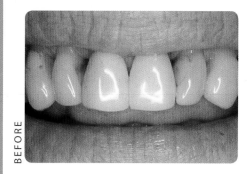

BEFORE

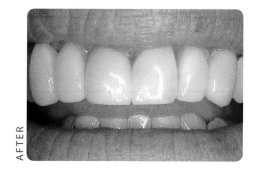

AFTER

10

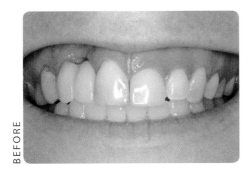

BEFORE

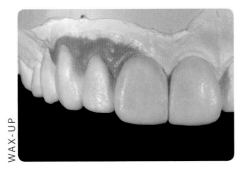

WAX-UP

You can't put a price on a beautiful smile » This attractive young woman had lost a tooth and was embarrassed to smile because of the resulting defect in the bone. Treatment included both bone and tissue grafts, crown lengthening, tooth extraction, implant placement, bleaching, porcelain veneers, an implant-supported bridge, and a fixed pink porcelain interdental addition to help mask any remaining deformity. This woman, like many other patients, felt it was well worth the investment of both time and money to have a great smile.

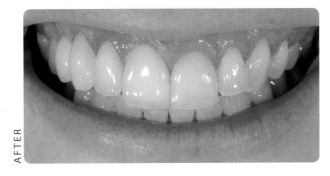

AFTER

WHAT CAUSES BONE LOSS?

When a tooth is lost or extracted as a result of gum disease or an accident, the bone around it heals at a slightly lower height than the tissue adjacent to it. In many cases, a bone defect results, making replacement with a fixed bridge difficult, if not impossible. Unless something is done to mask the defect, the teeth will look much too long. Three techniques that can be used to address the loss of bone are presented to the left.

---

smile 101 What are your options?

Fixed porcelain interdental addition	Removable artificial tissue appliance	Ridge augmentation
A fixed porcelain interdental addition is gum-colored porcelain (or composite resin) that is added to your bridge to mask the space between the restoration and the gum. The main challenge is obtaining a natural color match. Expect to pay about 25% more for a bridge with this special esthetic addition.	This appliance may be the easiest and least expensive way to mask missing gum tissue. It's made of flexible plastic, however, so it's fragile. It also requires maintenance. Cost of the appliance typically ranges from $450 to $1,500.	Ridge augmentation involves the addition of either transplanted or synthetic bone tissue to restore the ridge to its normal height. This surgical procedure allows the creation of a more esthetically pleasing and better-fitting fixed bridge.

what to eXpect

RIDGE AUGMENTATION

- **Treatment time:** One or more appointments of at least 1 hour
- **Maintenance:** Routine daily brushing and flossing as well as periodic professional cleanings
- **Results:** Replacement teeth appear to be naturally emerging from the gum tissue with no spaces or gaps
- **Treatment longevity:** Indefinite/long lasting
- **Cost:** Depends on number of teeth; usually $985 to $4,000

ADVANTAGES

- Can achieve a more esthetic, natural-looking result
- Makes it easier to clean gum tissue under bridge
- May improve speech
- Can help prevent trapping of food

DISADVANTAGES

- Lengthens treatment time
- Increases expense

10

If you have unattractive spaces at your gum line, consider having a

RIDGE AUGMENTATION

procedure before being fitted for a new bridge.

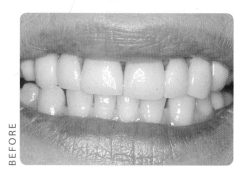

BEFORE

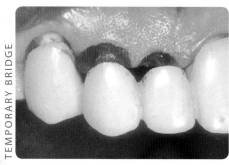

TEMPORARY BRIDGE

Give your new teeth long-lasting support » This woman disliked the unattractive spaces that showed when she smiled fully. The spaces were due to the loss of lateral incisors and canines, which resulted in bone and gum tissue loss around and between the missing teeth. Fitting of the temporary bridge revealed the extent of tissue loss. Ridge augmentation allowed for a more natural-looking fixed bridge that restored confidence to her smile.

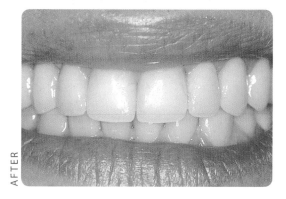

AFTER

What are your options?

Gingivectomy

A gingivectomy involves surgically removing some of the gum tissue. It is performed only if an adequate amount of attached gum tissue will remain.

Flap surgery

Flap surgery involves surgically lifting sections of the gum tissue so that the underlying bone and surrounding tissue can be treated. The flap is then reattached at a higher point so that less gum tissue shows when you smile.

Gingivoplasty

A gingivoplasty is a reshaping of the gum tissue. It can improve the contour of the gums around the teeth.

Orthognathic surgery

Orthognathic surgery involves removing a section of bone above the roots of the teeth and closing up the entire arch so that gum tissue is not visible when you smile. Although this is the most extreme and costly surgical alternative, if other procedures fail to provide the result you want, orthognathic surgery may be your best option (see chapter 11).

TIRED OF YOUR GUMMY SMILE?

For some people, too much gum tissue may be the result of disease, while others have inherited the tendency to have too much gum tissue. If gum disease is the problem, the overgrowth is usually thick and swollen and may bleed. This kind of inflammation is usually treated with scaling and curettage. If the problem is hereditary or the result of a high lip line, your dentist may suggest gingivectomy, gingivoplasty, flap surgery, or orthognathic surgery.

Good fit for good health » This young woman had crowns that did not fit properly, causing gum disease and the swelling shown here. Two new, well-fitting crowns were all that was necessary to clear up this woman's gum disease.

BEFORE
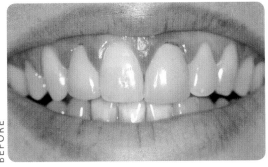

AFTER
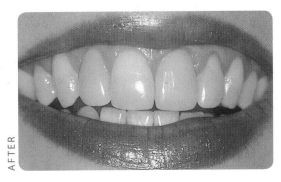

A new smile is a great investment » This woman was concerned about showing too much of her gums when she smiled. Her back teeth were not visible behind the poorly constructed crowns on the front teeth. The treatment plan included surgical removal of some gum tissue combined with new crowns that would be correctly proportioned and built out laterally to better fill out her smile. The result is a smile that still looks great 2 years after the cosmetic gum surgery and placement of the new crowns. Always invest in the finest ceramics to help achieve your most natural smile.

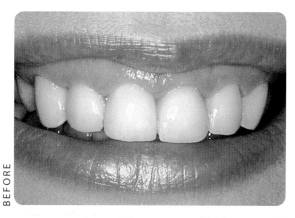

BEFORE

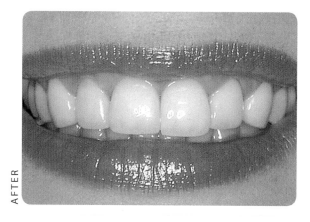

AFTER

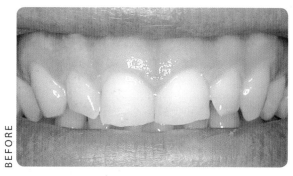

BEFORE

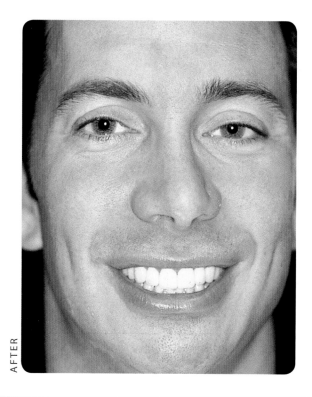

AFTER

Achieve the smile of your dreams » Big, beautiful, white teeth are what this man wanted most; instead, he had short, stubby, discolored teeth covered by a great deal of gum tissue. First, cosmetic gum surgery was performed. Ten weeks later, 12 porcelain veneers were constructed and placed, giving him the bright, white smile he'd always wanted.

10

A beautiful smile in one appointment » This 19-year-old student was dissatisfied with her existing plastic laminates and the way her gums showed when she smiled. The contour of the gum tissue was changed to be in harmony with her upper lip line, and 10 teeth were bonded with a lighter shade of composite resin in a single appointment.

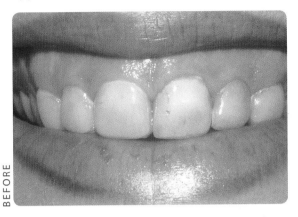

BEFORE

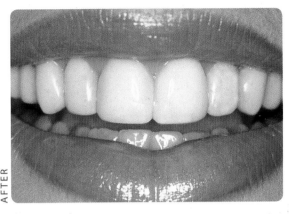

AFTER

Get rid of gumminess and stains for a whole new smile » This actress was displeased with her yellow teeth and gummy smile. The smile line was improved by surgically raising the gum tissue, and the teeth were bleached and then cosmetically contoured, creating a brighter smile.

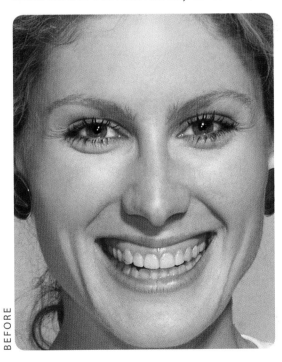

BEFORE

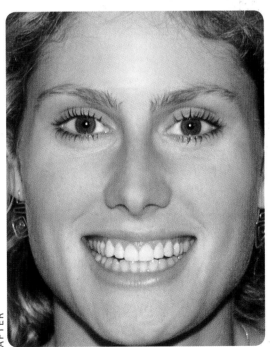

AFTER

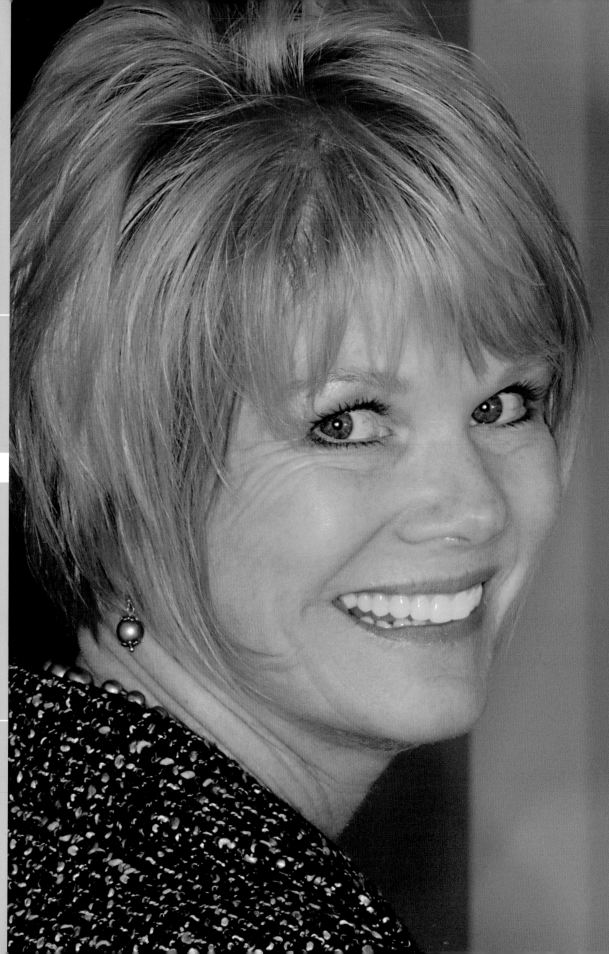

11

About Face

Louis S. Belinfante, DDS
Farzad R. Nahai, MD • Foad Nahai, MD

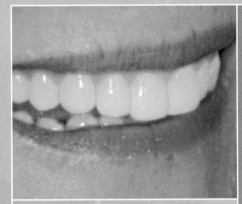

It may take more than a new smile to help you look your very best.

Having a great smile is undoubtedly an asset, regardless of other aspects of your appearance. However, your smile is only one part of the whole composition of your face. Once you have improved your smile, you may be inspired to make a few other changes to look your very best, and it may be necessary to look beyond your dentist for help.

If you are unhappy with your facial profile, the condition of your skin, or specific facial features such as your lips, nose, or chin, this is the chapter for you. In the first section, an oral and maxillofacial surgeon reveals how repositioning the jaws can improve not only your bite but also your entire facial appearance, especially in profile. The second section contains numerous hints and tips from plastic surgeons on how to get the most out of esthetic surgical procedures to enhance your facial features and overall appeal.

Orthognathic Surgery | Louis S. Belinfante, DDS

WHAT IS ORTHOGNATHIC SURGERY?

Orthognathic surgery involves dividing and repositioning the jawbones to bring them into better alignment. It is typically used to correct bite problems that cannot be fixed by orthodontics alone. Often bone or soft tissue may be removed or augmented to further enhance facial esthetics. Orthognathic surgery can bring about significant changes in your appearance, particularly as you are seen in profile.

IS ORTHOGNATHIC SURGERY RIGHT FOR ME?

Orthognathic surgery is typically performed by an oral and maxillofacial surgeon and can achieve dramatic improvement in facial esthetics. Orthognathic surgery may be the best option if you:

- Have jaw problems that can be treated only by surgery
- Can pay for the procedure or have adequate insurance coverage
- Feel strongly that your condition is inhibiting your success and happiness
- Are willing to experience some discomfort and inconvenience
- Understand and accept all associated risks

expert tip | Communication is critical to success!

- It's important that you tell your doctor exactly what you want to correct. He or she may zero in on a particular problem, and you need to be sure that problem is also your primary concern.

- Your surgeon will design a highly specialized treatment plan for you based on information gathered by obtaining casts of your teeth, photographs, video images, and special x-rays.

- It's highly important that you know what results to expect from treatment. Some surgeons will use digital imaging to give you a good idea of what you'll look like after surgery; others may show you tracings of your new profile based on your x-rays.

- It's also essential that you understand each step of the surgical procedure that you're toundergo. The main risks and possible outcomes should be explained thoroughly, and it's then up to you to decide which procedures you wish to have performed.

11

WHAT CAN ORTHOGNATHIC SURGERY DO?

Problems that can be addressed using orthognathic surgery include:

▶ Recessive or protruding lower jaw and/or chin

▶ Chin that is too short, too long, or otherwise unattractive

▶ Open bite (teeth do not meet)

▶ Lower and/or upper jaw positioned to one side or a narrow arch

▶ Discrepancies in upper and lower facial height (gummy smile or lack of enough tooth or gums showing)

WHAT YOU SHOULD KNOW

WHAT DOES AN ORAL AND MAXILLOFACIAL SURGEON DO?

Oral and maxillofacial surgeons do more than just tooth extractions and jaw surgeries. If you're interested in cosmetic procedures to enhance the appearance of your face and neck, talk to your surgeon about including them in your overall treatment plan.

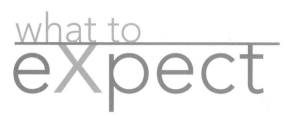

what to eXpect

HOW LONG DOES IT TAKE?

The actual operation may take from 1 hour to several hours, depending upon the complexity. Although some procedures require hospitalization for 2 or 3 days, the typical hospital stay is 1 to 2 days, and some orthognathic surgical procedures can be accomplished on an outpatient basis. If stabilization wire is used to keep the jaw in place, the wires will be removed in 3 to 8 weeks. If plates and/or screws are used, the time span for opening the jaws is much shorter. Your surgeon will then direct you back to your general dentist and orthodontist for the completion of treatment.

WHAT WILL I BE ABLE TO EAT?

If you require a hospital stay, you will probably be fed intravenously at first. However, as soon as you indicate that you can drink the liquids prescribed, the intravenous fluids will usually be reduced and then discontinued. You will probably experience some weight loss at first. However, a specific number of calories will be planned for you on a daily basis, and your diet will be supplemented with vitamins and minerals. As you regulate the calories you take in, your weight loss will level off.

IS IT PAINFUL?

Although you can expect some swelling and soreness, they are well controlled with medication. Because there are so many nerves in the mouth and facial area, there may also be some numbness after the operation. In most instances, normal feeling returns within a few weeks. When the wires are removed, you may experience some stiffness at first because the jaws will have been closed for a long time. After several weeks, however, you should be able to chew comfortably.

DOES SURGERY LEAVE SCARS?

Typically, the surgeon makes incisions from inside the mouth, chin, and cheeks so that there are no scars on the face. However, if screws and plates are used, small incisions in the skin may be necessary.

11

Taking shape » This 30-year-old woman was unhappy with the shape of her nose, and her chin did not fit her facial proportions. Surgery involved nasal and chin recontouring with the aid of implants.

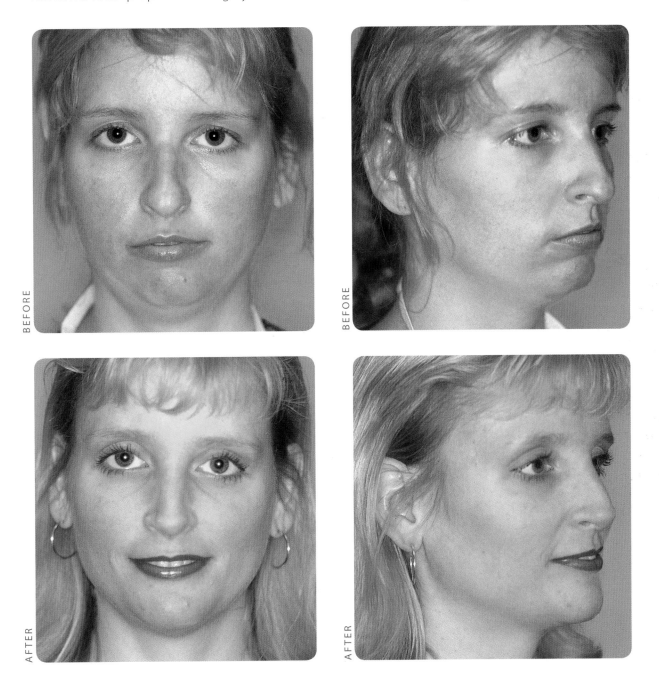

BEFORE

BEFORE

AFTER

AFTER

Research your surgeon!

- Make sure your surgeon is truly an oral and maxillofacial surgeon. He or she should be certified by the American Board of Oral and Maxillofacial Surgery and a member of organizations such as the American Association of Oral and Maxillofacial Surgeons.

- Find out what kind of training your surgeon has received.

- Try to obtain recommendations from other patients and/or other health care providers.

- Look up your surgeon on the Internet.

- Check to see at which hospitals your surgeon has privileges, and confirm that at least one of them allows the performance of the procedures in which you're interested.

- Ensure that your surgeon performs the procedure you're interested in on a regular basis.

- Ask to see before and after photographs of your surgeon's previous patients who have received the treatment you're considering.

- Take your time when discussing your treatment plan with your surgeon. Make sure you understand every aspect of the proposed surgery—don't be afraid to ask questions.

WHAT YOU SHOULD KNOW

FEES AND INSURANCE

▶ Costs for the initial phase of orthognathic treatment may range anywhere from several hundred to several thousand dollars. You should discuss fees before surgery takes place.

▶ If the procedures are performed for functional reasons, insurance may often cover hospitalization or clinic charges, as well as most of the surgeon's fees.

▶ Ask your doctor to write a letter to your insurance company that states the nature of your problem, the planned correction, and the fees involved. The letter should ask how much of the procedure will be covered.

ORTHODONTICS MAY BE REQUIRED

Many patients with jaw deformities also need orthodontic treatment to rearrange the teeth before or after surgery or both. In fact, it is almost impossible to obtain ideal results unless presurgical and postsurgical orthodontic therapies are performed.

Adjusting your alignment » The upper jaw of this 25-year-old man was positioned posterior to his lower jaw, causing his midface to appear sunken in and his upper teeth to be behind his lower teeth. In addition, the midlines of the upper and lower teeth were not aligned. He was also dissatisfied with the appearance of his nose, which had a deviated septum. Following orthodontic treatment, orthognathic surgery was performed to realign his jaws and correct his bite. Cosmetic surgery was also performed on his nose.

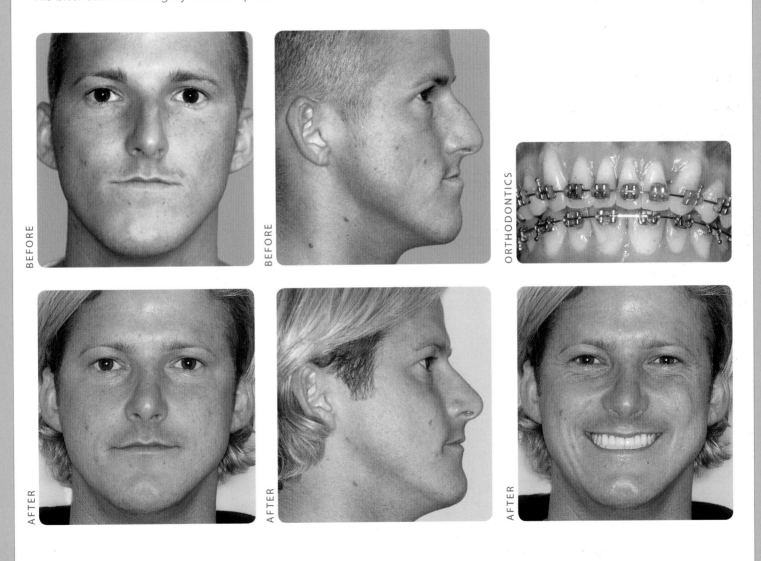

BEFORE

BEFORE

ORTHODONTICS

AFTER

AFTER

AFTER

Looking beautiful with orthognathic and cosmetic surgery » This 29-year-old woman had an open bite, a narrow upper jaw, and a recessive lower jaw and chin. She was also dissatisfied with the appearance of her nose and eyelids and the excess fatty tissue around her face and neck. Orthognathic surgery was performed to expand her palate, correct her open bite, and advance her lower jaw and chin. In addition, cosmetic surgery was performed on her nose and eyelids, and fat was removed from her face and neck.

BEFORE

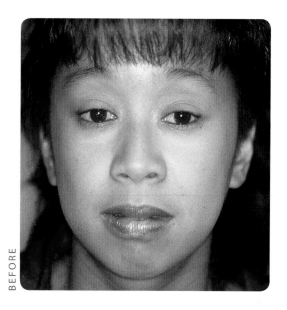

BEFORE

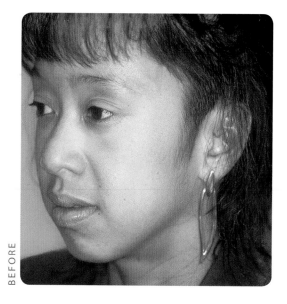

AFTER

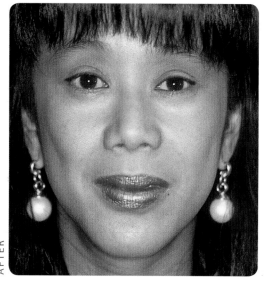

AFTER

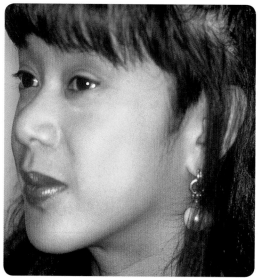

11

A growing problem » The upper jaw of this 16-year-old boy was too small for the rest of his face. Also, his lower jaw extended too far forward, and his chin was too short. In addition, he did not have permanent teeth coming in to replace 12 of his primary teeth. Treatment included orthodontics, prosthodontics, and oral and maxillofacial surgery. His upper jaw was advanced and vertically lengthened; the lower jaw was shortened; and his chin was lengthened both vertically and horizontally. After healing of the surgical sites, his primary teeth were removed and replaced by dental implants, on which bridges were placed.

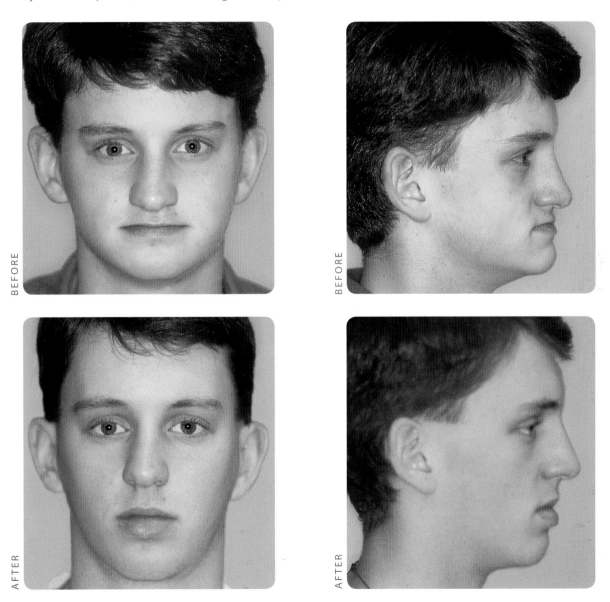

BEFORE

BEFORE

AFTER

AFTER

The beauty of symmetry » This 24-year-old woman had major facial asymmetry, mostly due to a bony protrusion on the left lower half of her face. This deformity also involved her upper jaw, lower jaw, chin, and bite plane. Surgery was performed to correct the unevenness of the upper jaw, and the lower jaw was surgically treated to match the new bite.

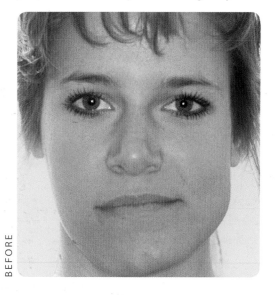

BEFORE

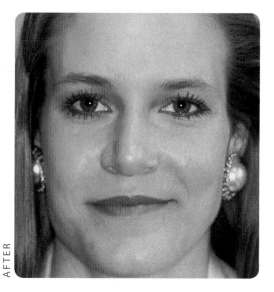

AFTER

Solving multiple problems in a single surgery » This 13-year-old girl had a retrusive lower jaw and chin, wide nose, and gummy smile. Following orthodontic therapy, in one surgery the lower jaw and chin were lengthened, the width of the nasal tip was decreased, and the height of the upper jaw was reduced to eliminate the gummy smile.

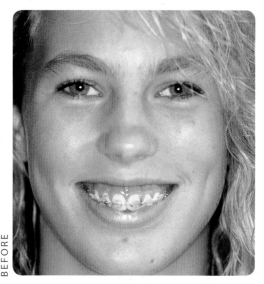

BEFORE

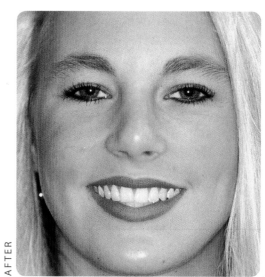

AFTER

11

WHAT WOULD YOU LIKE TO **CHANGE?**

This chart presents solutions for problems that are often corrected using orthognathic surgery and their related risks and estimated costs. However, fees will vary depending on the difficulty of the procedure; patient problems, history, and expectations; and the expertise of the surgeon. The recovery time for most procedures is several weeks, and the results are usually permanent.

PROBLEM	SOLUTION	RISKS	COST
CHIN DISCREPANCY	Surgery to reduce or increase chin height and/or move chin forward or backward, with or without implant placement	Nerve damage, swelling, bleeding, and infection	$3,000 to $5,000
SHALLOW CHEEKS	Cheek implants	Asymmetry, nerve damage, swelling, and infection	$4,000
PROTRUDING LOWER JAW	Jaw surgery and orthodontics	Nerve damage, altered bite, bleeding, and swelling	$6,000 to $8,000
OPEN BITE	Jaw surgery and orthodontics	Nerve damage, altered bite, bleeding, and swelling	$6,000 to $12,000
ASYMMETRY BETWEEN RIGHT AND LEFT SIDES OF FACE	Jaw surgery and orthodontics	Nerve damage, altered bite, bleeding, and swelling	$6,000 to $12,000
EXCESSIVE UPPER FACIAL HEIGHT	Jaw and possibly periodontal surgery, together with orthodontics	Nerve damage, altered bite, bleeding, and swelling	$6,000 to $12,000
REDUCED UPPER FACIAL HEIGHT	Jaw surgery and bone grafting	Nerve damage, altered bite, bleeding, and swelling	$6,000 to $12,000

Plastic Surgery | Farzad R. Nahai, MD **and Foad Nahai,** MD

THINK IT OVER!

There are good and bad reasons to have plastic surgery. Plastic surgery for the right reasons will be a satisfying experience. Plastic surgery for the wrong reasons will lead to dissatisfaction and disappointment. Take the quiz at right to determine whether plastic surgery may be a good choice for you.

ARE YOU A CANDIDATE FOR PLASTIC SURGERY?

Yes No

☐ ☐ 1. Do you think plastic surgery will add to your self-confidence?

☐ ☐ 2. Are you self-conscious about aging changes in your face?

☐ ☐ 3. Are you self-conscious about your nose?

☐ ☐ 4. Are you self-conscious about your chin?

☐ ☐ 5. Do you feel a more youthful appearance will be an asset in your job?

☐ ☐ 6. Do you think plastic surgery will bring about a significant change in your life?

☐ ☐ 7. Do you think plastic surgery will lead to a job promotion?

☐ ☐ 8. Do you think plastic surgery will alter a personal relationship?

☐ ☐ 9. Do you think plastic surgery will save a failing marriage?

☐ ☐ 10. Is your concern about the problems with your appearance out of proportion to what others think?

☐ ☐ 11. Are you looking for perfection?

Answering yes to questions 1–5 suggests that you have good reasons for considering plastic surgery. Answering yes to questions 6–11 suggests that you may have unrealistic expectations for plastic surgery.

11

WHAT YOU SHOULD KNOW

IT ALL STARTS WITH A GOOD SURGEON

A qualified surgeon is:

▸ Certified by the American Board of Plastic Surgery (www.abplsurg.org) or the American Board of Facial Plastic and Reconstructive Surgery (www.abfprs.com)

▸ A member of at least one of the major plastic surgery national organizations: the American Society of Plastic Surgeons (ASPS), the American Society for Aesthetic Plastic Surgery (ASAPS), or the American Academy of Facial Plastic and Reconstructive Surgery (AAFPRS)

▸ Happy to answer your questions about his or her qualifications

▸ Performing the procedure you're interested in on a regular basis with good results

You can find a good surgeon by:

▸ Asking someone who's had good results with esthetic surgery for the doctor's name

▸ Getting recommendations from your dentist or other physicians

▸ Visiting the websites of the ASPS (www.plasticsurgery.org), the ASAPS (www.surgery.org), or the AAFPRS (www.aafprs.org)

▸ Consulting with a second surgeon if necessary

▸ Requesting before and after photos of previous patients

Safety considerations:

▸ Your surgeon should be practicing in a facility certified by the American Association for Accreditation of Ambulatory Surgery Facilities (AAAASF), the Joint Commission on the Accreditation of Healthcare Organizations (JCAHO), the Accreditation Association for Ambulatory Health Care (AAAHC), or the American Osteopathic Association (AOA) or, in Canada, the Canadian Association for Accreditation of Ambulatory Surgery Facilities (CAAASF) and have privileges with at least one hospital in your community

▸ If you'll be under general anesthesia (fully asleep) during your procedure, an anesthesiologist must be involved in your care

Cosmetic surgery is not for women only!

Currently only about 10% of esthetic surgery is performed on men; however, the number is increasing as it becomes more acceptable for men to actively improve their appearance. Esthetic surgery on men is more challenging, partly because scars are more difficult to conceal because of shorter hairstyles and a reluctance to use cosmetics. However, most men are quite satisfied with the results and, like women, enjoy an emotional boost following surgery.

Nosing around » This young man broke his nose while playing sports and had undergone nose surgery, but his nose remained crooked, and he had difficulty breathing. In one outpatient operation (septorhinoplasty), the patient's breathing problem was corrected, and the appearance of his nose was improved. He is shown 1 year after surgery. Straightening the nose improved the overall symmetry and appearance of this man's face.

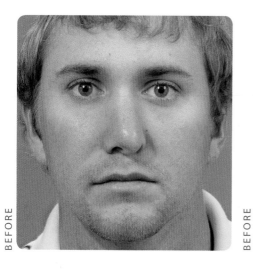
BEFORE

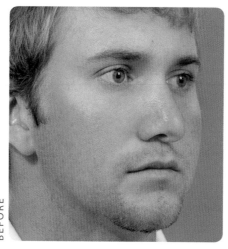
BEFORE

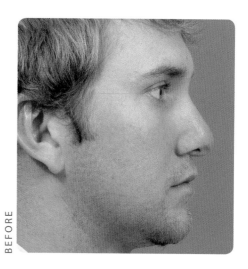
BEFORE

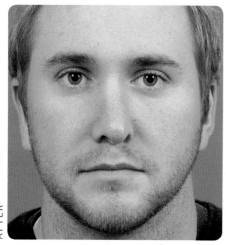
AFTER

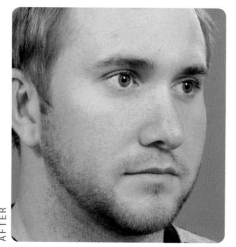
AFTER

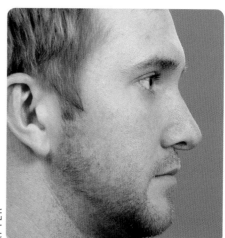
AFTER

11

When is the right time to have plastic surgery?

For correcting congenital deformities, age is not necessarily an issue. Cleft lip and palate should be corrected in infancy. An extremely large nose or other inherited features may be cosmetically corrected through plastic surgery at any time in the teen years or later. However, for diminishing the negative signs of aging, customizing over time is recommended. This means having minor procedures performed over time as they seem necessary. Each procedure will freshen your appearance gradually, making you the most attractive you can be at each age level. You don't want people to declare, "Look at that face-lift!" A subtle and gradual approach to cosmetic surgery elicits comments like, "You look so well-rested," or "Did you change your hairstyle?"

Sometimes less is more!

The most desirable results are achieved through subtle surgical correction. For example, with rhinoplasty, the nose need not be radically redesigned for the best results. The size and shape of the nose should be in proportion with the size and bone structure of the face. With facial esthetic surgery the goal is often a "younger" or "improved" version of yourself, not a radical transformation to look like someone else entirely.

WHAT YOU SHOULD KNOW

A VERY PERSONAL DECISION

Having a facial feature that deviates from common standards of beauty isn't reason enough to seek plastic surgery. A friend or loved one may suggest that you consider plastic surgery, but the ultimate decision rests with you. Remember, some of the most famous faces in the world have unconventional features, and yet these people, who could've easily afforded cosmetic surgery, decided against it. Conversely, if you desire plastic surgery and a qualified surgeon has confirmed that your expectations are reasonable and attainable, don't allow others to dissuade you.

Be open to suggestions!

In most cases your surgeon will agree with your assessment about which of your facial features can be enhanced through plastic surgery. However, he or she may suggest a different approach than you had in mind for a more desirable result. There is a wide variety of surgical and nonsurgical minimally invasive procedures available to enhance your smile and facial appearance. A thorough evaluation and consultation is essential to enable your surgeon to assess your particular needs, take into account your desires, and recommend the procedures and techniques that will produce the best possible results.

Raising your face value » This young woman was interested in improving the shape of her nose and having fuller lips. She first underwent surgery to reshape her nose (rhinoplasty), then had a brief in-office procedure to place filler into her upper and lower lips. Photos were taken 1 year after surgery. Note the improved overall facial symmetry after the rhinoplasty, which makes her eyes a more prominent feature in her face.

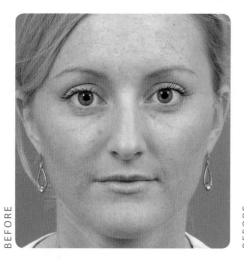

BEFORE

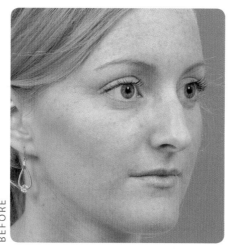

BEFORE

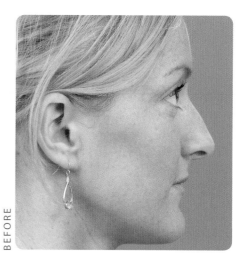

BEFORE

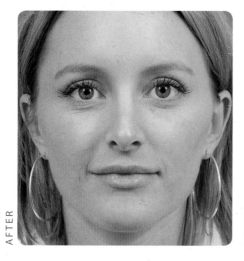

AFTER

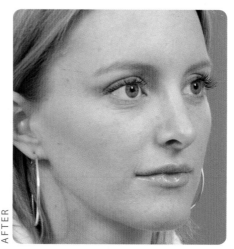

AFTER

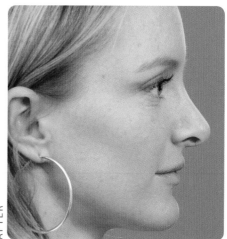

AFTER

11

WHAT YOU SHOULD KNOW

INJECTABLES: AN ALTERNATIVE TO SURGERY

While significant and long-lasting changes in appearance can be achieved with surgery, it's not the only option available to improve your appearance. Injectable products such as Botox and myriad other facial fillers are excellent options to minimize the appearance of facial wrinkles or plump the lips and cheeks. The advantage of injectables is that they're minimally invasive (all are done with a needle) with a very brief recovery time and almost instant results at a fraction of the cost of surgery. However, almost all injectables have to be readministered after a period of time to maintain the result. Be wary of any injectable that is permanent. It's very difficult to know how a permanent product will behave in the face over time.

Get your fill » This woman didn't like the uneven and deflated look of her face. She was interested in nonsurgical, minimally invasive ways to improve her appearance. Over the course of two office visits, Botox was administered to her forehead and brows, and facial fillers were placed in her lips and lower face. Note how robust and rejuvenated the patient appears, as well as the overall improvement in facial symmetry.

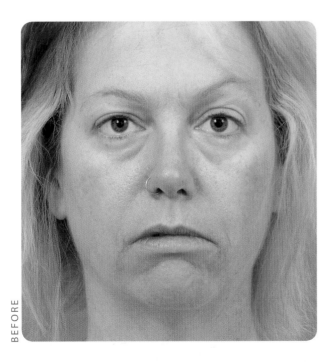

BEFORE

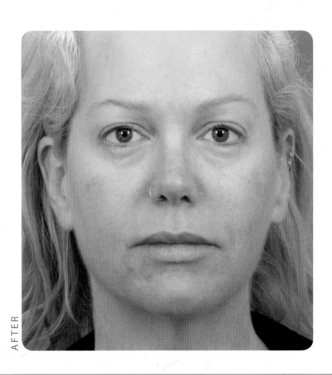

AFTER

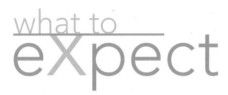

what to expect

COSTS OF SURGERY

The costs for facial plastic surgery may range from $1,000 for a minor procedure such as fat or filler injections to around $14,000 for a full face-lift. In addition to these costs, you may also have to include the cost of the hospital or clinic's surgical facility, as well as the fee for the anesthesiologist. You should feel comfortable inquiring about all of the costs before you decide to proceed. Esthetic surgery is not covered by insurance, and it is usual and customary for the surgeon's fee to be paid in advance.

smile 101 Do you really need surgery?

The plastic surgeon is an advisor who helps patients make good decisions. In some cases this means that a surgeon advises against surgery. Insecurity precipitates many people's desires for unwarranted plastic surgery. However, being advised against a specific cosmetic procedure may provide a boost in self-esteem for the person who's told by an expert that his or her concern is unwarranted.

WHAT YOU SHOULD KNOW

COSMETIC CLAIMS THAT SEEM TOO GOOD TO BE TRUE USUALLY ARE!

There have always been a wide variety of products and treatments on the market that make extraordinary claims that are simply not true. The confusing issue for the consumer is that many of these products are widely advertised and slickly promoted, which tends to make them seem legitimate. In many cases the procedures or products are unproven and have not been scientifically evaluated. The best way to ascertain the credibility of such products is to verify their effectiveness with a qualified medical professional. Also be wary of hype related to a particular surgeon, especially when someone is claiming to be the "best" or "only" person performing a certain procedure.

11

Give yourself a lift » This woman complained of looking stern and older than she felt. She wanted to look younger in her face. An endoscopic brow-lift, upper eyelid surgery (blepharoplasty), face-lift, and neck-lift were performed. Note the relaxed and more open appearance of her brow and eyes. She appears less stern and much younger.

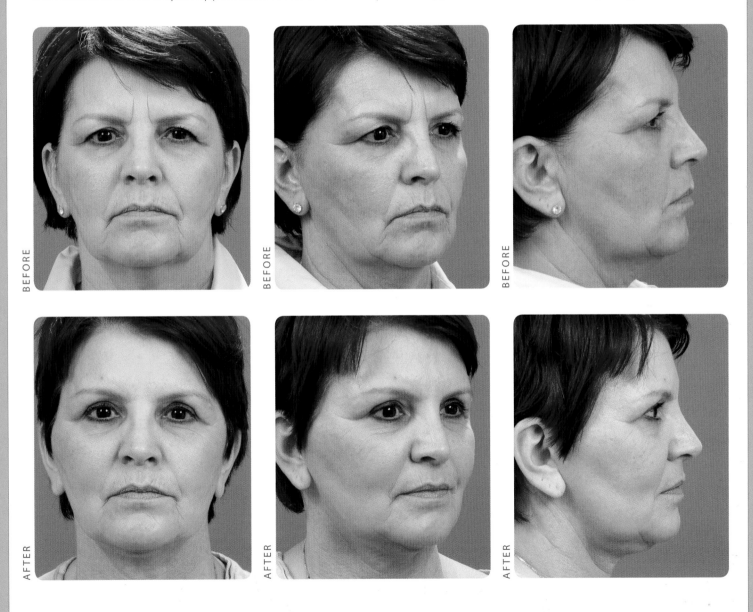

BEFORE

BEFORE

BEFORE

AFTER

AFTER

AFTER

expert tip Use topical treatments for healthier, younger-looking skin!

- Alpha hydroxy acids and Retin-A are effective in reducing fine lines and improving the general appearance of the skin, although they cannot eliminate established deep wrinkles.

- Electrical stimulation of facial muscles may produce temporary improvements in the appearance of skin.

- Moisturizing creams can improve, smooth, and protect the skin.

- Proper cleansing and daily skin care maintenance enhance the results of plastic surgery.

- Sunblock applied daily will help minimize the damaging effect of the sun on your skin over your lifetime, especially if you have fair skin or are often outdoors.

- Facial masks may be helpful for deep cleansing.

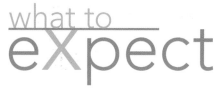 what to eXpect

GIVING INFORMED CONSENT

Before your surgery, you'll be asked to sign an informed consent form that will clearly state the general risks involved in any surgery as well as the specific risks that may be associated with your particular procedure. It may also detail such information as likelihood of success, practical alternatives, and prognosis if surgery is rejected. Rest assured that if you've done your homework and selected a qualified surgeon, he or she will recognize any complications that occur and be prepared to handle them successfully.

6 QUESTIONS TO ASK YOUR PLASTIC SURGEON

1. What will it do for my smile?

2. What are the risks?

3. What is the recovery time?

4. How long will the results last?

5. What will it cost?

6. What are the alternatives?

11

You won't believe your own eyes! » This woman complained that her eye area had an angry, heavy, and tired look. Upper and lower eyelid surgery (blepharoplasty) opened up the appearance of her eyes, making her look years younger. She is shown 5 months after surgery.

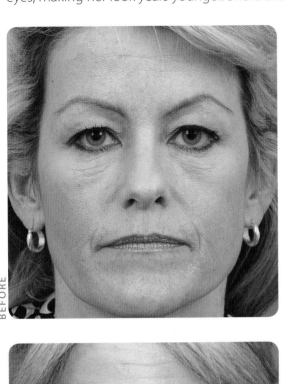

BEFORE

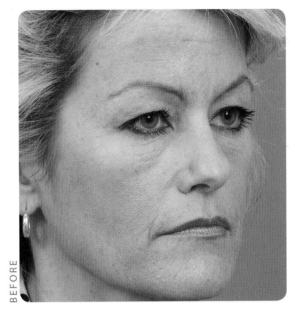

BEFORE

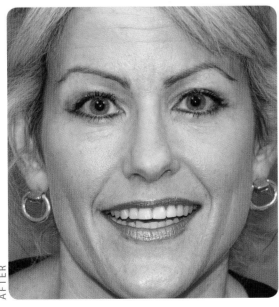

AFTER

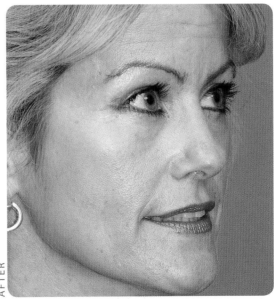

AFTER

WHAT WOULD YOU LIKE TO **CHANGE?**

PROBLEM	SOLUTIONS	RISKS
THIN LIPS		
	Lip augmentation using injectables or fat transfer	Temporary minor swelling and bruising
WRINKLED LIP AREA		
	Chemical peels and/or dermabrasion or laser resurfacing	Scarring and some discoloration, but these are minimal with the lighter peel
LAX, HEAVY, OR WRINKLED CHEEKS		
	Rhytidectomy (face-lift) liposuction, and/or buccal fat pad excision	Infrequent and usually minor; can include hematoma, facial nerve injury (rarely permanent), infection, and reactions to anesthetic; increased risk in smokers
NOSE TOO BIG, TOO LONG		
	Rhinoplasty (surgery to reshape the nose)	Infrequent and usually minor; can include infection, nosebleed, reaction to anesthetic, and small burst blood vessels that appear as tiny red spots on the skin's surface
PROTRUDING CHIN		
	Chin reduction	Bleeding, scarring, and nerve damage
BAGGY UPPER AND LOWER EYELIDS		
	Blepharoplasty (eye-lift)	Infrequent and usually minor; can include infection, reaction to anesthetic, double or blurred vision, temporary swelling, slight asymmetry in healing, and, rarely, inability to close your eyes
LOOSE NECK, EXTRA SKIN, OR FAT		
	Neck-lift and/or liposuction (often done with a face-lift)	Hematoma and minor skin irregularities that can be easily smoothed out
FROWN LINES, LAXITY, AND DROOPING BROW		
	Brow-lift	Altered ability to raise your eyebrow on one or both sides
FLAWED FACIAL SKIN		
	Chemical peel, dermabrasion, or laser resurfacing	Complications are extremely rare; can include infection, numbness, permanent skin color changes, and scarring

11

The chart on these pages outlines the most common facial esthetic problems and the procedures used to address them. It's intended to give you a general idea of what you can expect from treatment. Note that risks, results, and fees will vary depending on the specific circumstances of the patient and the surgeon.

RECOVERY TIME	TREATMENT LONGEVITY	COST
Overnight for injectables; up to 1 week for fat transfer	4–6 mo with injectables; much longer with fat transfer	$500 to $2,000
Depends on degree of treatment; 2–3 weeks	Generally considered very long lasting but depends on the depth and degree of treatment	Chemical peels and/or dermabrasion, $500 to $1,500; laser resurfacing, $1,000 to $2,000
Staged recovery; usually back to work in 10–14 days, almost all swelling and bruising gone by 4 weeks	Your face will continue to age, but the effects of the face-lift are everlasting. Avoiding sun and stress and maintaining good health will extend the effects.	Full face-lift, $8,000 to $14,000; buccal fat pad removal, $1,000 to $2,000; liposuction alone, $2,000 to $3,500
Staged recovery; usually back to work in 7–10 days, but limited strenuous physical activity for 2 weeks, and 80% of the bruising and swelling gone within 2 weeks	Results are permanent.	$2,000 to $5,000
2–3 weeks if bone is involved	Results are permanent.	$2,000 to $5,000
After 7–10 days may be able to conceal remaining bruises with makeup. Avoid strenuous activity for 2–4 weeks	Results last for many years and may even be permanent.	Both upper and lower eyelids, $3,000 to $6,000; upper or lower eyelids only, $2,000 to $4,000
For liposuction, minimal; for neck-lift, several weeks	Results will be permanent if weight and health are maintained.	Neck-lift, $3,500 to $5,000; liposuction of neck, $1,200 to $2,500
7–10 days with the endoscopic method	10–15 years	$3,500 to $5,000
Phenol peel: Return to work in 2–3 weeks; full healing in 3–6 months *TCA or glycolic acid peel and dermabrasion:* Recovery time much quicker (about 1 week). *Laser:* Variable depending on the type of laser used	Results are longer lasting with the phenol peel and dermabrasion than with the TCA peel and laser.	*Dermabrasion, lasers, TCA, and phenol peels:* full face, $1,000 to $3,000; regional, $500 to $1,500 *Glycolic acid and other alpha hydroxy acids,* $500 to $1,500

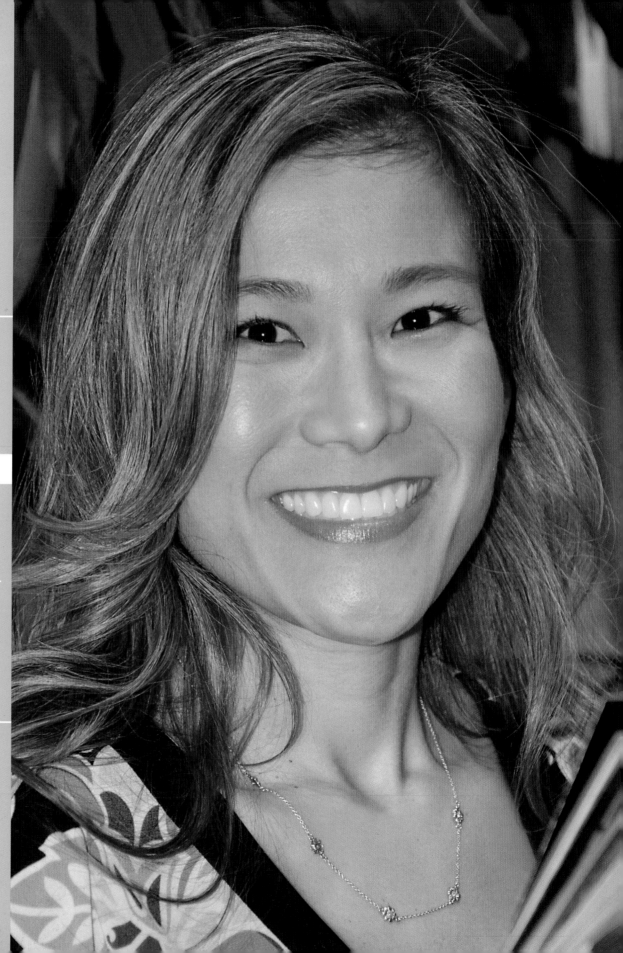

12

FIND OUT . . .

SECRETS TO MAKING YOUR
NEW SMILE LAST

HOW TO GET THE MOST OUT
OF YOUR SMILE

PROFESSIONAL TIPS FOR
LOOKING YOUR BEST

Finishing Touches

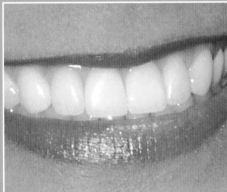

So you've got a gorgeous new smile. Now what?

Once you have the smile you always wanted, it's important to take care of it so it stays healthy and beautiful. The effects of most cosmetic dental treatments won't last forever, but you can make them last much longer by following the tips in this chapter.

Also, remember that a great smile is only the first step toward a whole new you. If you've been unhappy with your smile, you may not have taken the time to address other aspects of your appearance that could be improved. A new smile often brings the confidence and desire to make the most of what you've got. In addition, you may notice other things you want to change that you didn't see before because you were so distracted by flaws in your smile. The cosmetic procedures presented in chapter 11 may be the best solution for some problems, but others may be easily addressed using the tips provided by beauty and hairstyle experts in the second part of this chapter. You won't believe the difference a few small adjustments can make in your appearance, confidence, and outlook on life.

BREAK THOSE BAD HABITS!

If bad habits ruined your smile in the first place, they'll spoil your beautiful new smile as well if you don't break them. For example, smoking and drinking excessive amounts of coffee and tea will stain your restorations or newly bleached teeth. Grinding your restored teeth and chewing on or holding hard objects between them can cause wear, gaps, and chips or fractures that may stain. Be sure to discuss all past and present habits with your dentist, and remember, if you want your new smile to last as long as possible, you'll need to leave your old bad habits behind.

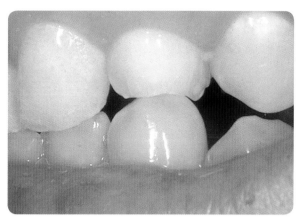

Grinding can ruin your new teeth »
A side-to-side grinding pattern destroyed the beautiful shape of this patient's canine.

IS YOUR HABIT PUTTING YOUR NEW SMILE IN DANGER?

Do you now or did you ever:

Yes No

1. Chew, bite, or suck your lips or cheeks?
2. Suck your fingers or thumb?
3. Chew ice?
4. Bite your fingernails?
5. Hold pins or needles in your mouth?
6. Chew pencils or pens?
7. Chew or hold your eye-glasses in your mouth?
8. Crack nuts with your teeth?
9. Drink more than three cups of tea and/or coffee per day?

Yes No

10. Smoke a pipe, cigars, or cigarettes or use chewing tobacco?
11. Keep your tongue pressed against the upper teeth?
12. Place your tongue in a space between your teeth?
13. Grind or clench your teeth?
14. Vomit after eating to lose weight?
15. Take methamphetamines or other habit-forming drugs?

12

expert tip Save it for later!

Restorations have limited life spans, and it's necessary to replace them periodically. Each time this is done, a little more tooth structure may be lost. For this reason, conservative treatment is encouraged early on, particularly in young people. The best advice is to ask your dentist if your restoration could be sealed and reinforced instead of replaced.

WHAT YOU SHOULD KNOW

7 SIGNS YOU NEED TO REPLACE A RESTORATION

1. It's discolored, and you find it esthetically unappealing.

2. It has cracks or chips, and the remaining tooth structure isn't protected.

3. It's no longer fitting well or is "leaking."

4. It's showing signs of wear. (If too much wear occurs, filling material will no longer support the enamel.)

5. You're experiencing sensitivity. (The cement may have washed out or the margins may be faulty.)

6. Your dentist tells you that the restoration isn't compatible with your gum tissue.

7. There are microcracks adjoining the restoration.

KEEP YOUR **SMILE BEAUTIFUL!**

Ask your dentist at every checkup if any of your restorations are showing signs of wear. If they are, do something about it sooner rather than later. Keep in mind that your restorations are made to support your enamel, so when they wear, your enamel may fracture. Worn restorations may also lead to discoloration and loss of tooth contour. Most restorations remain in place long after they begin to fail, and many patients grudgingly accept the resulting problems as inevitable— but they aren't!

YOU ARE WHAT YOU **EAT**

Ultimately, beauty emanates from good health, and good health begins with proper nutrition. Be sure your diet includes a proper mix of fresh vegetables and fruits, whole grains, and lean protein, and drink plenty of water daily. What you put into your body is reflected in your skin tone, nails, hair, tooth structure, and in your overall sense of well-being.

 expert tip **Give your smile a healthy frame!**

Overeating or undereating can change the shape of your face. This, in turn, can alter the proportion of your tooth size to your face, thereby affecting your smile. To keep your smile looking its best, maintain a healthy weight through exercise and a balanced diet.

Second chance for a beautiful smile » This 34-year-old interior designer suffered from bulimia for 15 years, which caused severe erosion and tooth sensitivity. After 2 years of therapy to control her eating disorder, the patient wanted to restore her smile. Ceramic crowns were placed to help relieve tooth sensitivity and enhance the patient's smile. A beautiful smile can go a long way in improving the self-image of a person who has had an eating disorder.

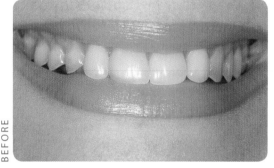

BEFORE

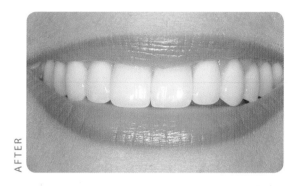

AFTER

WHAT YOU SHOULD KNOW

EATING DISORDERS ARE DANGEROUS

Too many times, emotional problems are reflected in our eating habits. Psychological stress or trauma can cause people to overeat or develop eating disorders like anorexia and bulimia. These conditions not only wreak havoc on emotional and physical health but may also cause serious damage to your smile. For example, bulimia can cause severe dental erosion, destroying the beauty of teeth. This erosion causes loss of enamel, resulting in the exposure of dentin (the darker layer underlying the enamel). If you have an eating disorder, no amount of cosmetic dentistry or plastic surgery will correct it. Seek professional help for the underlying problem. Gaining determination and confidence can have a tremendous impact on your self-image. You can then turn your attention to your appearance and do what it takes to keep your smile looking its best.

12

expert tip — A bigger smile is a better smile!

Practice smiling with your mouth open and teeth showing. A square or round face can appear longer or more oval when the mouth is in a more open position. Also, make sure the bottom biting edges of your upper teeth are visible. Opening the mouth a bit more may keep the lower lip from covering the edges and prevent the teeth from looking like a row of Chiclets gum. If these tips work for you, practice them in front of a mirror so that when you smile naturally, you'll know subconsciously how much to open your lips. This procedure is especially effective for photographic purposes.

Show the edges of your teeth! » A smile that shows only the surfaces of your teeth is not as appealing as a more open smile. Note how this man's smile appears more attractive with the biting edges of his upper teeth visible. Smiling this way takes conscious effort, however, so it's a good idea to practice it until it becomes second nature.

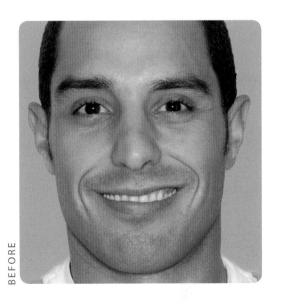

BEFORE

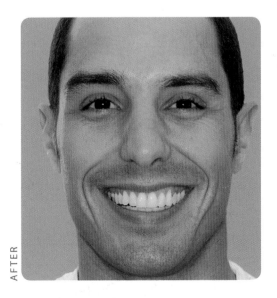

AFTER

USE YOUR NEW SMILE!

Many people who've had corrective dental treatment forget that their smile looks better. If, for example, you've spent years hiding your mouth with your hand whenever you laughed or smiled because you were embarrassed by your teeth, it will probably take conscious effort to break yourself of the habit. When you complete your cosmetic dental treatment, practice smiling in front of a mirror. Think of something funny so that you really reveal your teeth. Repeat this until you get used to smiling again. Then remember to smile often—it increases your face value!

A smile looks best when it's surrounded by smooth, clear skin. Proper skin care is most effective when you make it an integral part of your morning and evening rituals. In the morning a good skin care routine is invigorating, and at night it provides an excellent opportunity for relaxation. This isn't just about slowing the aging process, being attractive, and having self-confidence; it's also about spectacular physical, mental, and spiritual health and fitness. Caring enough about yourself to include your health and beauty needs in your schedule gives you the opportunity to heal, reorganize, refresh, and decompress or re-energize.

15 SECRETS TO HAVING CLEAR, HEALTHY SKIN

Environmental and hormonal factors play a role in breakouts and skin sensitivities, but you can improve your chances for great skin by doing the following:

1. Choose an appropriate skin care regimen, and use it twice a day (once in the morning and once before bedtime).

2. Use an appropriate facial mask, and exfoliate at least once a week.

3. Take showers when you bathe.

4. Wash your face *after* using shampoo and conditioner.

5. Apply all skin care products before hygiene or hair care products.

6. Keep your skin care containers clean and free of dust so that you don't pick up irritants from the outside of the bottles.

7. Brush and floss your teeth before cleansing your face. The bacteria-laden plaque between your teeth can cause blemishes and irritation if it lands on your face and neck.

8. Don't let aerosol products settle on your back, shoulders, or face.

9. Keep your hands away from your face during the day, and be sure to clean the telephone receiver before using it.

10. If you have to touch your face, wash your hands first.

11. Don't pick or squeeze a blemish—this will only worsen the problem. Instead, apply an appropriate blemish treatment, then leave it alone.

12. Use a clean pillowcase every night until the breakouts and sensitivity stop. The hair care products and natural oils in your hair may be causing the problem.

13. Be aware that exposure to the sun, wind, chlorine, cigarette smoke, and smog can cause or worsen a breakout or sensitivity.

14. Use a sunscreen for sensitive skin only during the daylight hours—such products tend to be drying to the skin.

15. A good self-tanning product provides a safe and natural-looking tan year-round. Be sure to use a specially formulated facial self-tanner on your face.

12

Get that healthy glow! » Having healthy, clear skin can dramatically improve your overall appearance and provides a beautiful canvas on which your new smile can shine.

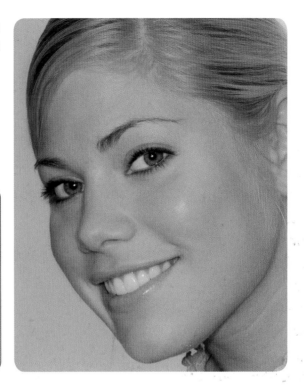

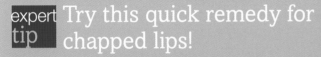 **Try this quick remedy for chapped lips!**

Apply a thick coat of lip balm to the lips extending over the edges, and allow it to remain there for a minute or two. Then using a moistened soft cloth buff the lip balm away with a gentle yet firm back and forth motion until the peeling skin comes off easily. Reapply the lip balm often to prevent future chapping.

smile 101 It's all in the lips!

The skin on the lips can easily get dry and chapped, and with age, it quickly loses its collagen, oil, and moisture. As a result, the lips droop and provide less support to the surrounding skin, promoting the formation of smile lines and wrinkles. However, there are some simple things you can do to achieve and maintain sumptuous, younger-looking lips:

- Apply lip balm daily. It's best to choose one with SPF 45 or higher. The lips are very sensitive to the sun and can even develop dark spots and freckles over time.

- Try using a lip balm that contains essential vitamins and nutrients to keep your lips moisturized and healthy. Some lip balms even have antioxidants to protect against the aging effects of free radical damage.

- If your lips are beginning to thin and age, try applying a lip mask once or twice a week. It will provide extra moisture and help to restore and smooth your lips.

- Avoid acidic or spicy foods when your lips are dry and chapped. Until they've healed, a better choice is hydrating foods, such as melons or cucumbers, which will actually cool and moisturize your lips.

Whether you're a man or a woman, the hair on your face can greatly affect the appearance of your smile. Of course, for women, unwanted facial hair can only detract from a great smile—the question is how to remove it without making a bad situation worse. For men, however, it's a bit more complicated. Deciding on a facial hair style—the clean-shaven look, a beard, a mustache, sideburns, or a goatee—is a very personal choice that depends greatly on your features and personality.

smile 101 To beard or not to beard?

- Generally speaking, if you had facial hair before getting your new smile, it's a good idea to at least try shaving it off afterward. Many people grow facial hair to hide or distract attention away from their smiles, but now you've got a great smile—show it off!

- If you have a receding chin or if the lower part of your face is asymmetric, think about growing a beard to help balance out these irregularities.

- Consider growing a mustache to create the illusion of better facial proportions if your chin is too prominent in comparison to the upper portion of your face.

- You may want to consider shaving or at least trimming your mustache if your teeth have been restored or bleached in a lighter color but still look dark. A mustache creates a shadow over the teeth, making them look darker.

- If you aren't happy with your current facial hair style or if you're just looking for a change, don't be afraid to try something different. The best (and worst) thing about facial hair is that it will grow back quickly!

- No matter what style your facial hair is, make sure it always looks neat and well groomed.

expert tip Seek professional help for your brows!

It's strongly recommended that you go to a professional for your first brow shaping or to correct previously misshaped brows. If you desire to continue to do your own brow upkeep, it's important to get professional brow shaping and grooming instructions. If you pluck out too many brow hairs from the wrong place, you run the risk of them not growing back as full or at all.

12

Some men look good both with and without facial hair, so their decision is best made based on the image they wish to project. This handsome young man had allowed his facial hair and his hair to grow while he was traveling, giving him a rugged look. After he shaved and got a much shorter haircut, his look was more updated and approachable. (Makeup by Rhonda Barrymore; hair by Richard Davis.)

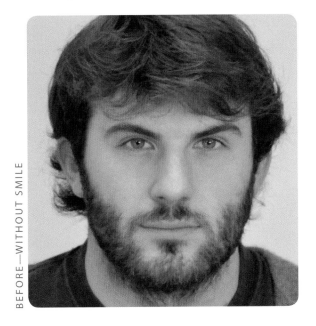
BEFORE—WITHOUT SMILE

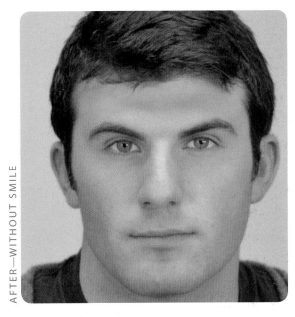
AFTER—WITHOUT SMILE

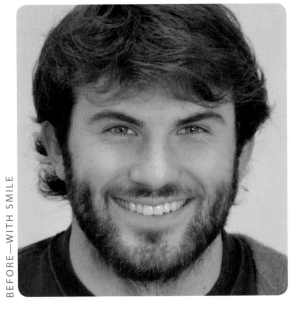
BEFORE—WITH SMILE

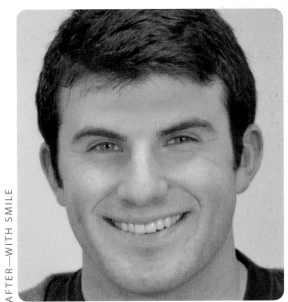
AFTER—WITH SMILE

WHAT YOU SHOULD KNOW

FACIAL HAIR REMOVAL TECHNIQUES

Professional methods:

▶ Waxing

- Hot or cold wax is spread over the area, and a fabric strip is applied on top of it. The practitioner quickly snaps the strip away from the skin, removing the hair with the wax. The results of this type of hair removal last about 4 weeks.

- The area may become and stay red for several hours. Sunscreen should always be worn on the waxed areas to prevent sun damage, premature aging, and freckling.

- Repeated brow and lip waxing over many years can lead to sagging skin.

▶ Laser epilation

- This method uses light to get rid of dark, coarse hair on light skin. Lasers cannot remove light or very fine hair.

- Lasers create a quick pinching sensation and can cause a flare-up of acne and possibly discolor skin permanently.

- This technique usually requires six to eight sessions spaced at least 2 weeks apart. The results are long lasting, but not permanent.

▶ Cosmetic electrolysis

- A practitioner uses a tiny probe with an electric current and sometimes chemicals to destroy the hair matrix cells in each hair follicle.

- This is the only system currently deemed by the FDA to provide permanent hair removal.

- Electrolysis is considered painful and can be a long and costly method of hair removal.

▶ Threading

- This is an ancient hair removal system in which a practitioner winds cotton thread around his or her fingers in a crisscross pattern and moves it swiftly across the facial skin with a scissor action, plucking and shearing hairs along the way.

- Regular trips to the salon are required to keep the skin hair free. Be aware that even skilled threaders can accidently cut the skin.

12

Do-it-yourself methods:

▶ Razor shaving

  – It's a myth that shaving causes hair to grow back thicker. Shaving with a razor with multiple wire-wrapped blades, shave gel or oil, and aftershave products provides an inexpensive and quick solution to unwanted facial hair.

  – If you have a persistent thick hair on your chin area, shave the fragile tip off first and allow it to surface overnight, then pluck it.

  – Occasional gentle exfoliation of the shaved areas will prevent ingrown hairs from forming.

  – For shaving the brow area, use a brow razor with a wire-wrapped blade, and place your index finger on top of your eyebrow to prevent accidental removal.

▶ Electric shaving

  – Shaving with an electric razor provides the same results as above, but you'll want to use a shaving powder instead of a gel or oil.

▶ Tweezing

  – By using precision tweezers at the correct angle and with a little practice, you can quickly and easily remove coarse hair from the face by plucking each hair one at a time.

  – This method is not recommended for men's beards, although a man can use it to lightly groom his brows.

  – Tweezing is long lasting because the hair is removed from the root, and it's a great way to remove facial hair between professional hair removal appointments.

  – Occasional gentle exfoliation of the tweezed area will prevent ingrown hairs from forming.

▶ Electronic epilator

  – This battery-operated handheld system features a rotating barrel-shaped head with tiny tweezers that open and close randomly to provide quick and easy facial hair removal for days to weeks.

  – The first use may be as painful as waxing, but with continued use the pain subsides.

  – These tiny devices do not remove cells from the epithelium of the epidermis and are therefore one of the safest ways to remove hair.

▶ Chemical depilatory

  – This is a quick and inexpensive method for facial hair removal, but use caution: The chemicals can cause irritation and burns if left on the skin too long.

ENHANCE
YOUR NATURAL BEAUTY

Although it shouldn't be confused with an everyday must like skin care, makeup is a fabulous fashion accessory and mood elevator. Color cosmetics can be applied to accentuate your best features, disguise imperfections, and highlight your gorgeous new smile.

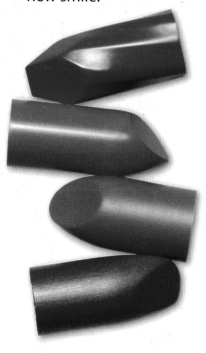

HOW TO APPLY NEUTRAL COSMETICS FOR EVERDAY ELEGANCE

1. Before applying makeup, make sure your skin is clean and moisturized.

2. Apply a moisturizer or moisturizing concealer to your eyelids.

3. Apply a matte eye shadow in a shade that matches your skin color on the eyelid from just above your lashes to the crease of the eyelid, from corner to corner, with a wide eye shadow brush.

4. With a rounded shadow brush, apply matte eye shadow in a medium shade to the eyelid crease, extending slightly above the indention. Blend well.

5. In the outer corner of the eyelid just below the crease, apply a slightly deeper shade of matte eye shadow over the base color and up slightly over the color in the crease. Blend the edges together with a clean brush.

6. Apply a soft shimmer eye shadow in a color slightly lighter than your skin color to the outer edge of the brow bone and up to the brow line, then blend.

7. Apply a tiny amount of brow powder in your appropriate shade to the brows for shape and definition.

8. Line your top eyelids with a waterproof crème liner or a soft pencil liner in a deep shade.

9. Use an eyeliner brush to apply a soft eye shadow color to the lower lid line.

10. Curl your lashes and apply waterproof mascara, allow it to dry, then apply a second coat.

11. With your fingertips, add a small touch of crème blush to the apples of your cheeks, extending to the upper area of the temples.

12. Apply a pressed mineral powder in your skin's natural color over the crème blush and to the entire face with a small kabuki brush. Apply evenly, blending at the neck area.

13. Apply a hint of pressed powder matte blush to the center part of the apples of your cheeks, and blend slightly to the edge of and over the crème blush with a soft blush brush.

14. Finish your face with a pressed invisible blotting powder to ward off shine.

15. Follow with an appropriate lipstick color. You can top it off with a sheer lip lacquer for longer wear and a glossier lip color.

12

Show off your new smile with beautiful lips!

- When selecting a lipstick shade, try one that matches the color of your gums exactly. It will more than likely make your teeth look whiter and become a favorite lipstick that you'll go back to over and over.
- Choose a shade of lip liner that matches your lip color. Don't apply liner (or lipstick) outside the border of your lips.
- Deep matte colors make lips appear thinner and older, whereas shimmery colors give lips a fuller and younger look.

MAKING UP THE DIFFERENCE

This woman has a heart-shaped face, so the goal of the makeover was to balance her narrow chin with the width of the upper part of her face. The makeup artist applied a crème foundation lighter than her natural skin tone as a highlight on her chin to diminish its sharpness. She then softened her forehead and cheek areas with darker shades of powder and blush. The hairstylist gave her hair long layers to add fullness around her chin line and just a wisp of bangs to give her a more balanced look. The split image demonstrates the dramatically positive effect makeup alone can have. (Makeup by Rhonda Barrymore; hair by Richard Davis.)

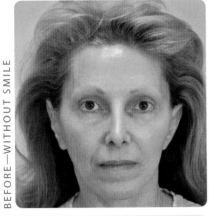

BEFORE—WITHOUT SMILE

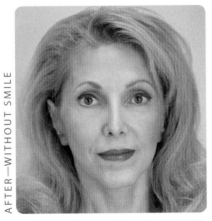

AFTER—WITHOUT SMILE

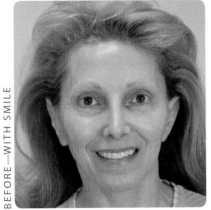

BEFORE—WITH SMILE

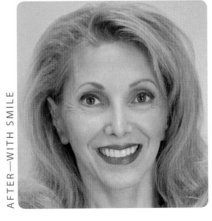

AFTER—WITH SMILE

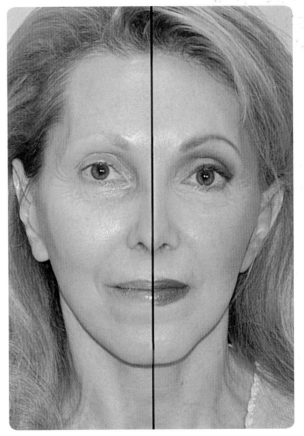

207

No one has a perfect face; even after you've improved your smile and perhaps undergone other cosmetic procedures, you'll still have some features that are better than others. Therefore, it's important to choose a hairstyle that complements your good features and minimizes the negative ones. The best way to achieve this is to find a hairstyle that balances your facial shape. The most pleasing facial shape is oval, so the goal is to use your hair to bring your facial shape as close to that ideal as possible. If you have a short face, your hairstyle should lengthen it; if you have a long face, a style that shortens it a bit will work best.

expert tip — Try a new hairstyle risk-free!

If you're a bit squeamish about trying out a brand-new hairstyle or just unsure what cuts might work best for you, try going online to sites that allow you to see how different styles will look on you. The digital previews and expert advice on the following pages were provided by TheHair-Styler.com, an interactive site that allows you to upload your own photos and try out different virtual hairstyles. It also provides a free hair consultation, articles on hair trends and tips, and photos of celebrity hairstyles for inspiration. The more you can tell your stylist about what you want, the better your chances of getting a hairstyle you'll love.

No hair necessary! » Rather than struggle with a receding hairline, many men choose to shave their head. This look can be pulled off successfully if you've got good facial structure and a great smile to support it. You can see how a bright new smile made all the difference for this world-class Tai Kwan Do champion.

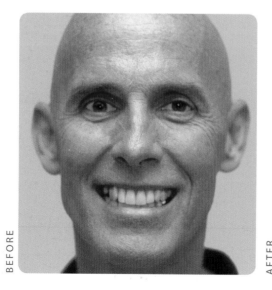

BEFORE

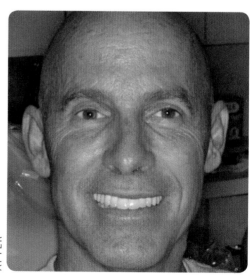

AFTER

12

ROUND FACE SHAPE

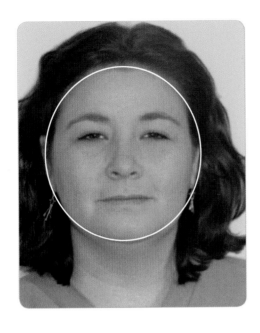

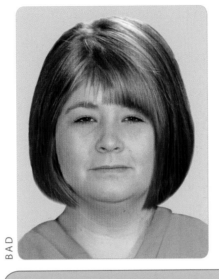

BAD

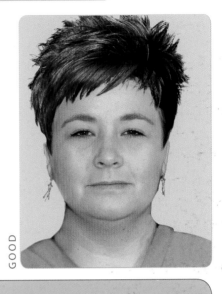

GOOD

If you have a round–shaped face . . .
You will want to choose a style that adds height to your face, but no width. Short haircuts often work best. If you prefer a medium or longer style, choose one with a middle part and little to no volume on the sides. Avoid side parts and long, heavy bangs that are cut straight across, as these will shorten your face further. (Hairstyles courtesy of TheHairStyler.com.)

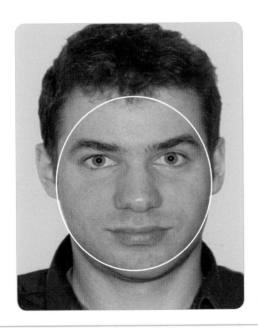

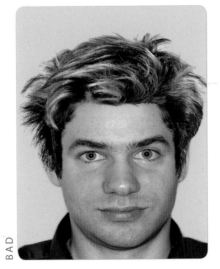

BAD

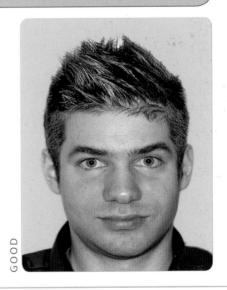

GOOD

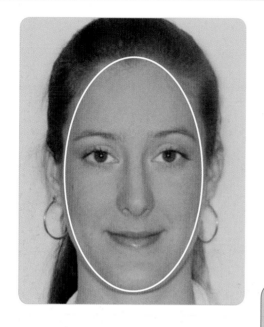

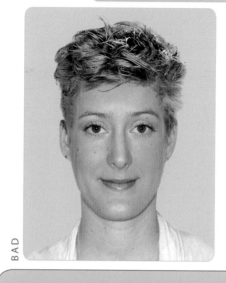

BAD

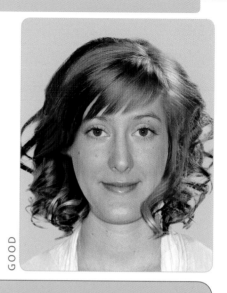

GOOD

If you have an oblong–shaped face . . .
The main objective is to reduce the length of the face, which is best accomplished by increasing the width. Styles with side parts and long bangs cut straight across work very well. Adding body with waves and curls also helps to soften and shorten the appearance of an oblong face. Avoid middle parts and styles that are full on top or have no body or bangs. (Hairstyles courtesy of TheHairStyler.com.)

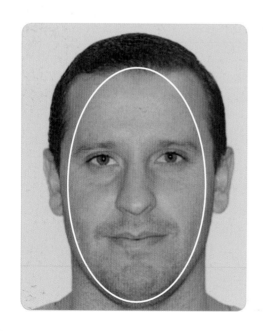

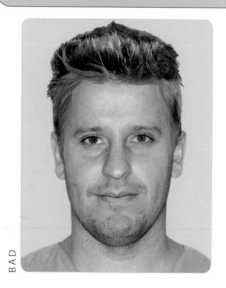

BAD

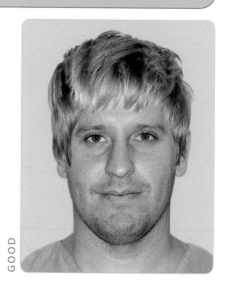

GOOD

12

SQUARE FACE SHAPE

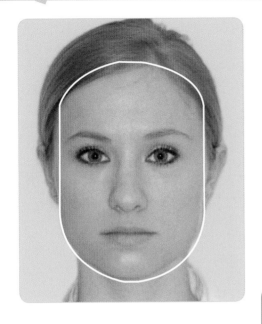

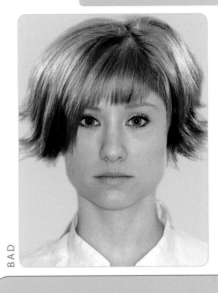

BAD

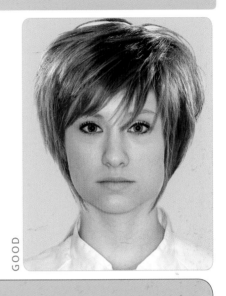

GOOD

If you have a square–shaped face . . .

Look for styles that will de-emphasize the squareness of your jawline, such as rounded or wispy cuts and bangs that sweep to one side. Avoid any cuts that create a straight line, particularly chin-length styles and middle parts with solid bangs. (Hairstyles courtesy of TheHairStyler.com.)

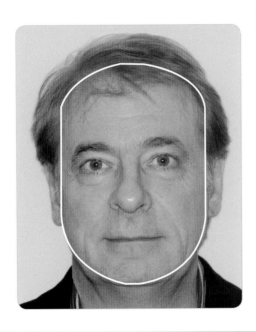

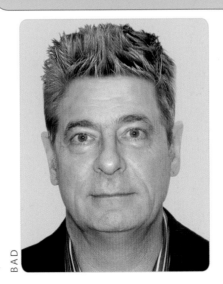

BAD

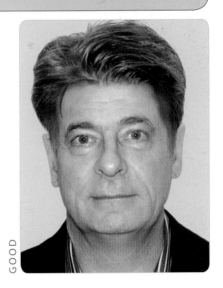

GOOD

211

HEART FACE SHAPE

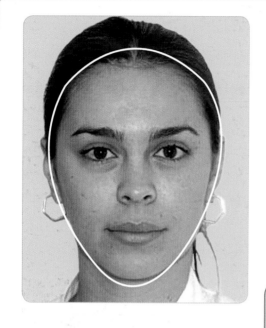

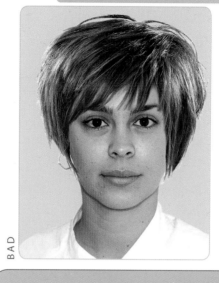

BAD

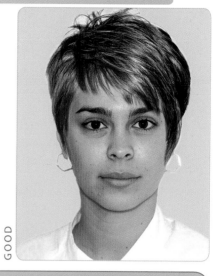

GOOD

If you have a heart–shaped face . . .

It is best to choose a cut with height on top to reduce the width of your forehead and draw attention away from your narrow chin. Styles with texture and layers work best, particularly if they are cut to chin length. Any cut that will increase the width of your upper face should be avoided. These include short, full cuts and long, heavy bangs cut straight across. (Hairstyles courtesy of TheHairStyler.com.)

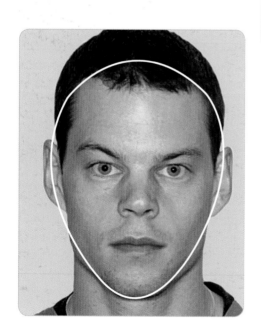

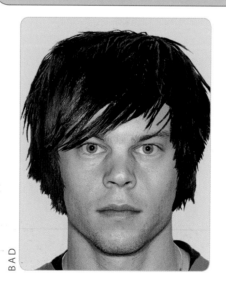

BAD

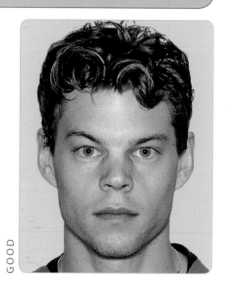

GOOD

12

OVAL FACE SHAPE

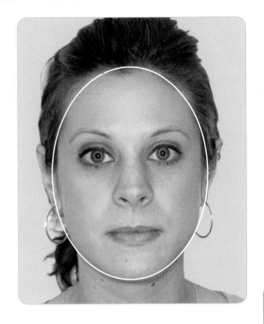

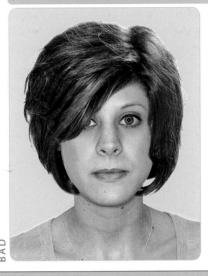

BAD

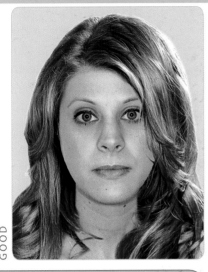

GOOD

If you have an oval–shaped face . . .

You've got the ideal facial shape, which means your options are wide open. The only guidelines are to choose styles that accentuate your best features and don't cover too much of your face. It's also best to avoid cuts that add too much width to your face, which can make a perfect oval face appear too round or square. (Hairstyles courtesy of TheHairStyler.com.)

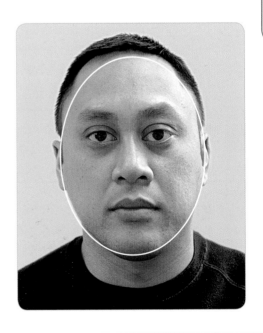

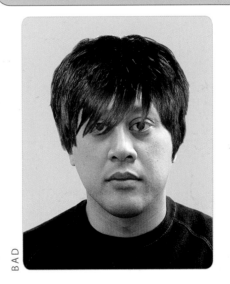

BAD

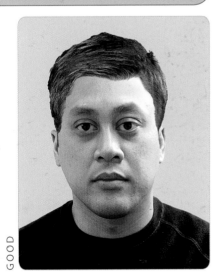

GOOD

APPENDIX

HOW IT'S DONE

This appendix offers you a quick study of the major cosmetic dentistry techniques presented in this book. Take a few minutes to read about the solutions suggested for your particular problem so you can better understand the procedures your dentist may recommend. The more knowledge you obtain prior to your consultation, the better able you'll be to ask specific questions and make the best decision for your smile.

Bonding

Bonding with composite resin was introduced approximately 50 years ago. The tooth enamel is gently etched to enhance adhesion before a dentist applies color-matched resin compound over a stained, crooked, short, chipped, decayed, or broken tooth. A special light is then used to harden and bond it to the tooth underneath. The composite resin is then contoured and polished to look like natural enamel.

HOW DOES **BONDING** WORK?

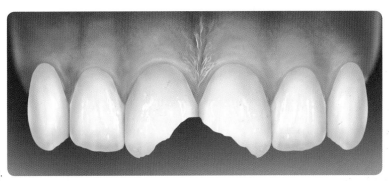

Fractured teeth prior to bonding.

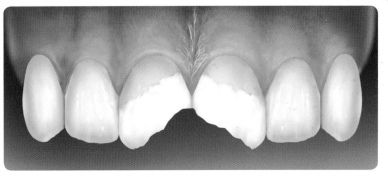

The enamel has been etched in preparation for the attachment of the composite resin.

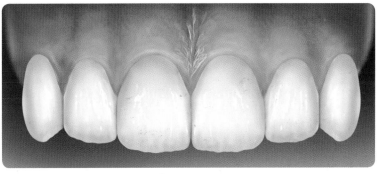

Composite resin has been applied. Bonding is painless and can usually be accomplished in one appointment.

Porcelain Veneers

Natural-looking, strong, and stain-resistant, wafer-thin porcelain veneers can be used on just one or multiple teeth to improve the appearance of a crooked, discolored, worn, or chipped smile. To create perfect fit and adhesion, your dentist most likely will need to reduce the thickness of the teeth, then chemically etch the enamel before placing the veneers. The beauty of porcelain is that it resists staining and can even strengthen the tooth when bonded correctly.

HOW IS A **PORCELAIN VENEER** PLACED?

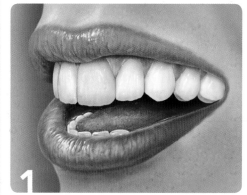

1 A porcelain veneer will be placed on the stained left central incisor.

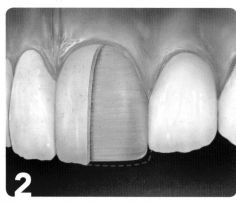

2 The enamel is reduced to help make room for the veneer. Once reduction is complete, an impression of the prepared tooth is made so that the porcelain veneer can be constructed in the dental laboratory.

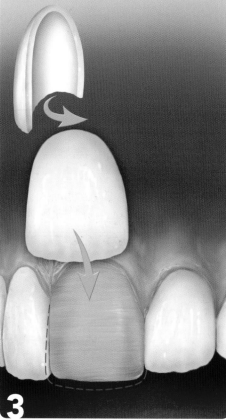

3 The remaining enamel surface of the tooth and the inside portion of the veneer are etched and coated with a resin cement, then the veneer is placed on the tooth.

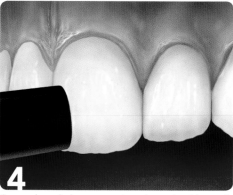

4 Once placed, the veneer is polymerized (cured) by high-intensity light for a few seconds.

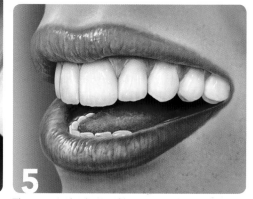

5 The veneer looks just like a natural tooth, and the surrounding tissue is healthy.

ENAMEL REDUCTION WITH VENEERS

If porcelain veneers are your treatment of choice, you and your dentist must decide whether or not to remove enamel from the front surfaces of the teeth, and if so, how much. The purpose of reducing enamel is to make room for the veneer.

ADVANTAGES

1. Less chance the tooth will look too bulky.
2. Better tooth form usually means better gingival health.
3. Greater chance for successful esthetic result.

DISADVANTAGES

1. The procedure is generally not reversible.
2. The tooth may appear darker as more enamel is reduced because the underlying dentin is darker than the enamel.
3. The more enamel removed, the greater the likelihood of a problem with the tooth pulp.

Turn back the years with porcelain veneers » This former beauty queen was unhappy with her smile. She wanted to recapture the look she had when she was younger. She brought several photos of herself at a younger age to her initial appointment, and computer imaging was used to give her an idea of the results she could expect. She now once again has an award-winning smile.

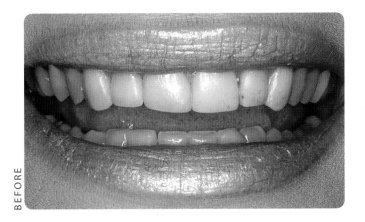

BEFORE

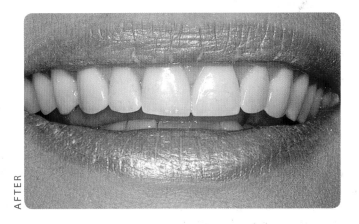

AFTER

Crowns

A full crown is a 360-degree replacement of the tooth enamel as well as some dentin. Also called *caps,* crowns can be used to make a crooked smile appear straighter or to repair broken or damaged teeth. A crown also can be placed on an implant to replace a missing tooth. Crowns often are used side-by-side with veneers in a full-mouth restorative treatment.

HOW IS A **CROWN** PLACED?

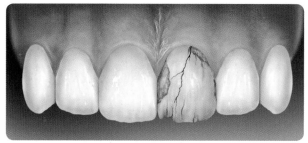

The tooth is severely fractured and chipped, making placement of a crown the best treatment alternative.

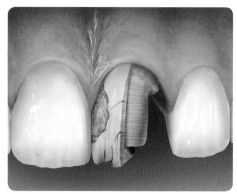

Half of the tooth has been prepared, showing the approximate amount of tooth structure that has been removed.

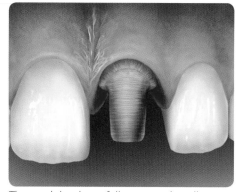

The tooth has been fully prepared to allow space for the porcelain (and often an underlying layer of metal for support).

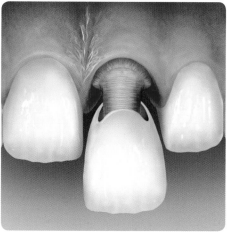

The new crown is placed. Notice how it will fit up under the gum tissue to hide the margin (junction) between the natural tooth and the crown.

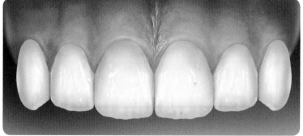

The final crown is shaped to look and feel natural then is attached with special dental cement. The esthetic goal is to make the crown appear as if it's naturally emerging from the soft tissue.

PINS VS POSTS

Fractures often leave teeth weak and in need of support. In such cases, a pin or a post can be placed in the tooth to provide added strength and create a core around which to build a restoration.

PINS
- Sometimes are used in back teeth to add retention for filling materials
- Typically aren't used with composite resins
- May be cemented, tapped, or screwed into place to add support when nerve removal is unnecessary
- Generally cost from $100 to $350 each

POSTS
- Often are placed inside a tooth when the nerve has been removed
- Are used if significant chewing force will be exerted on the crown and there's limited tooth structure remaining
- Typically cost from $250 to $650 each

TYPES OF CROWNS

There are several types of esthetic crowns. Some are made entirely of high-strength porcelain or cast glass; others combine metal and porcelain. The type of crown you and your dentist choose will depend on a number of factors, including the location of the tooth or teeth being crowned, the severity of the problem, and the overall health of the surrounding gums. Let your dentist advise you on which type of crown will be best in your particular situation.

METAL-CERAMIC WITH WITH ALL–METAL MARGIN

ADVANTAGES
- Strongest
- Least expensive

DISADVANTAGES
- Metal may be visible if tissue shrinks or is thin
- Metal may affect color of ceramic

METAL-CERAMIC WITH PORCELAIN BUTT JOINT

ADVANTAGES
- Esthetic
- No metal shows from front
- Strong

DISADVANTAGES
- Metal usually visible when mouth is wide open
- Metal may affect color of porcelain in rare cases
- Margin more susceptible to chipping
- More expensive to fabricate

ALL-CERAMIC

ADVANTAGES
- Most esthetic throughout crown life
- No metal shows

DISADVANTAGES
- Not as strong as metal-ceramic crown
- Margin may be more susceptible to chipping
- More expensive to fabricate

HOW TO MAKE THE MOST OF YOUR ESTHETIC TRY-IN

▸ Avoid use of an anesthetic if possible so that your lip line can be seen in its natural condition.

▸ Ask for a large mirror that shows your entire face, and hold it at arm's length to get an idea of how your smile is seen by others.

▸ Look at the restorations from various angles and in different types of lighting using natural expressions.

▸ Don't make split-second decisions. Look at the restorations long enough to grow accustomed to them.

▸ Consider your dentist's opinion as well as your own.

▸ If there's someone whose opinion you value highly, be sure to bring him or her with you to the try-in.

▸ Above all, be honest. If you aren't happy with what you see, now is the time to make necessary changes.

COMMUNICATION IS ESSENTIAL

You may be asked to sign a written statement of approval when you're satisfied with your appearance at the try-in appointment. Treatment shouldn't progress until you, your dentist, and anyone else involved are pleased with the appearance of the restorations. However, it's important to keep in mind that once the teeth are ready for a try-in, it may be too late to make radical treatment changes. If you want a particular "look," be sure to discuss it with your dentist from the start.

TEMPORARY CROWNS CAN HELP YOU DECIDE

Usually your dentist will provide you with temporary crowns made of either acrylic or composite resin while final restorations are being made. These "temporaries" can help you become accustomed to having a new color and shape in your mouth if teeth are being lengthened or if a new bite is formed. They also can help you decide—in advance—if you like what you see and if you want to make any changes. If you'll be wearing temporaries for any length of time, consider paying more for better ones. Although more esthetically pleasing temporary restorations take longer to make and have a higher cost, the results are usually worth it.

YOU'LL HAVE TO GET USED TO YOUR CROWNS

Your new restorations will not feel normal overnight. Your tongue, cheeks, lips, and brain need time to adjust, which typically takes a week or two, particularly if drastic changes have been made. Relax, and try to get your mind off your mouth. With a little time, you can grow accustomed to almost anything new. If your bite doesn't feel right, however, see your dentist immediately. If allowed to persist, a bad bite can cause pain and damage to the temporomandibular joints.

ESTHETIC CHECKLIST FOR YOUR NEW CROWN

Yes No

☐ ☐ **1. Does the color blend in with the rest of the teeth?**
The objective is to make the crown look as natural as possible.

☐ ☐ **2. Is it too long or too short?**
Ideally, the biting edges of your upper teeth should just touch the bottom lip when you say "forty-five." Remember, if you want a younger smile line, the two central incisors should be slightly longer than the two lateral incisors.

☐ ☐ **3. Does the gum tissue look healthy?**
It should outline each tooth in a half-moon shape. Red, puffy, or bleeding gums are unhealthy. Healthy gums have the texture of an orange peel.

☐ ☐ **4. Is the dental midline aligned with the facial midline?**
Ideally, an imaginary vertical line drawn between the two upper central incisors should be in line with the middle of the face. If not perfectly in line, it at least should be parallel to the facial midline.

☐ ☐ **5. Does the shape of the crown duplicate the form of the natural tooth?**
Bring an old photograph of yourself if you have one to help the dentist create the best form for you. Your tooth shouldn't be too bulky, and it shouldn't look like the gum is pushing it out of the mouth. It should slide right under and fit flush with the gum line.

☐ ☐ **6. Do the surface characteristics of the crown match those of the adjacent teeth?**
If your adjacent teeth have ridges or other irregularities on their front surfaces, your crown should also include these surface details so the light will reflect off the crown the same way as it does off the natural teeth.

☐ ☐ **7. Could the adjacent teeth be improved with cosmetic contouring or a new filling?**
Many times your results can be greatly enhanced by simply improving the shape of your adjacent and/or opposing teeth.

☐ ☐ **8. Does the tooth placement look natural?**
Sometimes the addition of a little porcelain or a slight reshaping can make a tooth look a bit irregular and more natural.

WHAT HAPPENS IF YOUR GUMS SHRINK?

CROWN TYPE

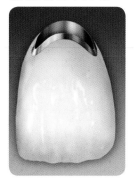

Metal-ceramic crown with all-metal margin.

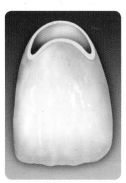

Metal-ceramic crown with porcelain butt joint.

All-ceramic crown.

GUM SHRINKAGE

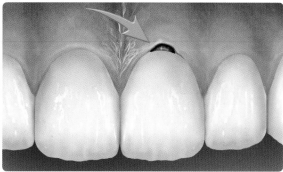

Exposure of the metal margin.

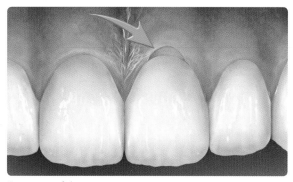

Exposure of the root.

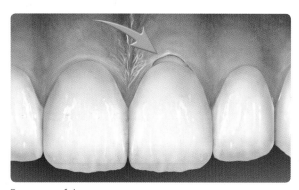

Exposure of the root.

REPAIR

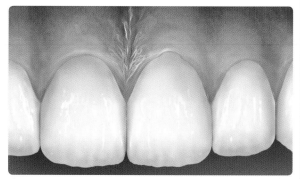

The metal margin is still somewhat visible following placement of composite resin.

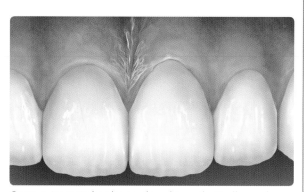

Composite resin has been placed to esthetically mask the root and blend in with the porcelain butt joint.

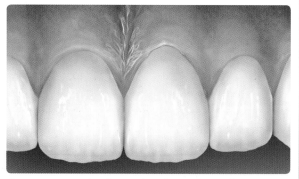

Composite resin has been placed to esthetically mask the root and blend in with the all-cermaic crown.

A SPARE SET MAY BE YOUR BEST BET

Because crowns invariably seem to break on weekends or during travel—never when it's convenient to see a dentist—it can be a good idea to have a backup.

If you're having porcelain crowns made, a spare set can be fabricated at the same time, usually at a lower cost. If budget constraints prohibit you from purchasing an extra set, consider keeping temporaries on hand as an interim fix. At the very least, ask your dentist either to save the mold from which your crown was made or give it to you to keep. Many times this mold can be reused, saving you the cost of new impressions.

ADVANTAGES

1. Less expensive than starting over.
2. You get instant replacement in case of fracture.
3. You can save the cost of a temporary or an extra office visit.
4. You could beat inflation; your crowns could cost more later.

DISADVANTAGES

1. Your initial cost is more.
2. You may never need the extra set.
3. Your tooth may change with time, causing the spare crown to not fit properly.
4. If your gum line changes around the neck of the tooth over the years, the spare crowns may be useless.

WHAT TO DO IF YOUR CROWN BREAKS

- See your dentist as soon as possible, particularly if your tooth is sensitive. The inside portion of the tooth may be exposed, or the tooth may be damaged, necessitating immediate treatment.

- If you aren't able to see a dentist immediately, continue to brush your teeth as usual, avoiding any sensitive areas. Otherwise, bacteria can build up and aggravate your problem. Then, see a dentist as soon as possible. Postponing treatment can result in additional damage.

- If you have a spare crown or temporary, use it to replace the broken one. Just don't neglect to get another spare to replace the one you're now wearing!

- If you don't have a spare crown or temporary, save the fractured piece of porcelain. Hopefully it can be bonded into place until a new crown is made.

- Don't attempt to repair the broken crown yourself. Some of the glues on the market can dissolve in your mouth. Moreover, if you use a cyanoacrylate-based glue, your dentist may not be able to separate the glue from the tooth in order to reposition the fractured piece more precisely.

Bridges

A bridge is a replacement of a missing tooth or teeth. A fixed bridge is cemented in place, whereas a removable bridge can be taken out for cleaning. A bridge can be retained by adjacent teeth or implants (see the next section). Although most fixed bridges have a metal substructure, all-ceramic bridges are now possible thanks to advances in ceramic materials. Once the bridge is constructed, your dentist will try it in so you can evaluate its fit, color, and size and make sure your bite is correct. Any necessary modifications can be made at this time, then reglazing or polishing is performed, and the bridge is cemented in place.

HOW A **CONVENTIONAL FIXED BRIDGE** WORKS

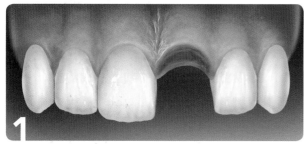

1 A conventional three-unit bridge will be used to replace the missing central incisor.

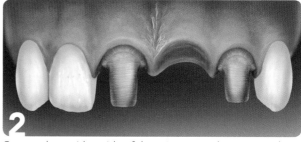

2 One tooth on either side of the missing tooth is prepared to retain the fixed bridge.

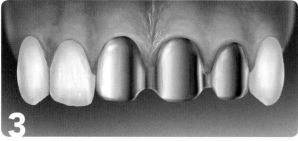

3 The metal framework of the bridge, to which porcelain will be fused, is tried in the mouth. All-ceramic frameworks are also available.

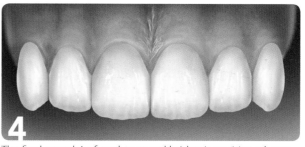

4 The final porcelain-fused-to-metal bridge is positioned over the teeth and just under the gum tissue to hide the seam between the porcelain and metal.

HOW A **RESIN-BONDED BRIDGE** IS ATTACHED

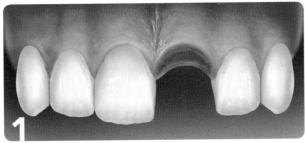

1 A resin-bonded bridge will be used to replace the missing central incisor.

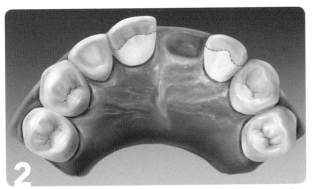

2 View of the roof of the mouth. The enamel on the backs of the two adjacent is reduced slightly.

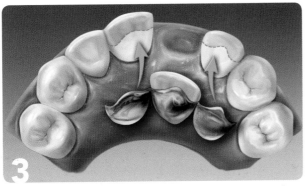

3 The backs of the teeth and the inside of the metal "wings" are etched. A strong composite resin cement is used to bond the metal to the teeth.

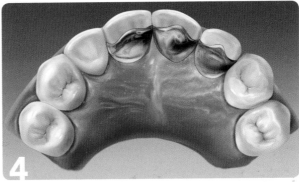

4 This inside view reveals how the strong and yet thin metal wings have now bonded the replacement tooth to the adjacent teeth.

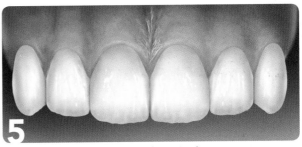

5 Notice how no metal is visible from the front.

Implants

One of the most exciting advancements in dentistry has been the dental implant. It's a natural-looking, usually permanent, secure way of restoring or replacing missing teeth that has allowed millions of people who have been unable to chew for years to regain the chewing ability of their youth. In most cases, implants are titanium anchor posts that are surgically placed in the jawbone and capped with a full crown or bridge.

HOW **IMPLANTS** ARE PLACED

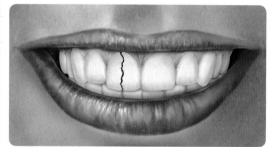

This fractured tooth requires extraction.

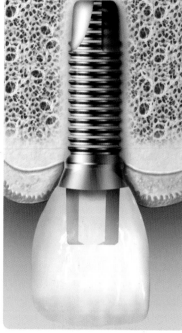

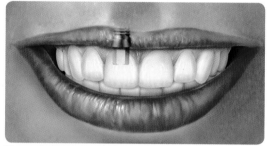

The superimposition shows the position of the implant in the final smile.

Appearance of the gums following tooth extraction.

Cross section showing the relationship of the implant to the bone and gums following surgical implant placement and attachment of a crown.

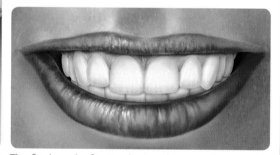

The final result after implant and crown placement is both functional and esthetic.

WHO CAN PLACE IMPLANTS?

Implant treatment is usually provided by a team including a surgeon (a periodontist or an oral surgeon) to place the implant, a dental laboratory technician to fabricate the crown, and a restorative dentist to place the crown. However, some general dentists are trained in implant dentistry and perform both the surgical and the restorative phases of treatment. Although implant dentistry is not a formal dental specialty, many practitioners have undergone extensive implant training, and some even limit their practices to implant treatment.

IMPLANT TREATMENT STEP-BY-STEP

Implant treatment can be immediate or take several months depending on your situation. Following are the basic phases and steps of treatment, although they'll vary based on your particular needs. The surgical phase is typically performed in two stages, although it can sometimes be done in one.

PRESURGICAL PHASE

- Your mouth is examined thoroughly, and x-rays of your head, jaw, and teeth may be taken. Today many dental surgeons use a CT scan, which provides the dentist with a 3-D look at the site where the implant will be placed. This can help the surgeon to plan where the implant will be placed into your bone with great precision.

- Impressions of your teeth and/or ridges are made to help the dentist determine exactly where the implants should be placed.

- Occasionally, blood tests as well as a medical examination may be required prior to implant placement to determine your overall health status and predict the success of treatment.

SURGICAL PHASE (TWO-STAGE SURGERY)

- An incision is made in the gum, the implant is placed, and the gum tissue is stitched back into place. This can be done with a local anesthetic in the dentist's office or under sedation or general anesthesia in a hospital or clinic. In certain patients, the implant can be placed directly in the bone without the need for incision.

- Following surgery, you'll probably experience some swelling and discoloration of the gums as well as some discomfort, which can be relieved with medication. Within a few days, the gums should return to normal. To allow the implants to heal properly, a soft diet is recommended for 4 to 6 weeks.

- The second stage of surgery is usually performed 2 to 6 months after the first in an outpatient setting. The dentist numbs the areas with local anesthetic, makes an incision in the gums to expose the implants, and connects abutments to the implants.

- The gums are stitched into place and a temporary restoration placed on the abutment. At times, additional gum surgery may be required for esthetic purposes. If you're missing all of your teeth, a comfortable dressing or your old dentures (relined with a soft material) will be placed over the abutments to promote healing and reduce discomfort.

- Impressions may be made so that the dentist knows where to position your new teeth.

- Your dentist should instruct you about how to keep the abutments clean.

POSTSURGICAL PHASE

- About a month later, your new teeth are fitted. In some cases, they're attached to a metal framework. In other cases, the artificial teeth may be attached to natural teeth or stand alone.

- Several checkups are scheduled during the following year so your dentist can ensure that your implants are functioning properly. After that, you'll need regular maintenance checkups. Follow-up x-rays are taken regularly.

HOW A **BRIDGE** IS PLACED ON **IMPLANTS**

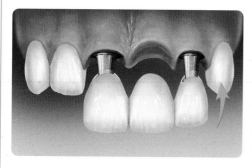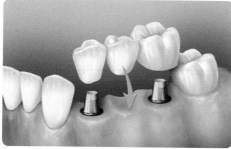

Shown here are three-unit all-ceramic bridges being placed on two implants in the anterior (*left*) and posterior (*right*) regions of the mouth. See the previous section for more information about bridges.

A NEW TOOTH IN ONE DAY

Immediate loading is an alternative way of placing implants in which the implant and the crown are placed in the same visit. This eliminates the need for a second surgical phase and greatly speeds up the implant placement process. If you have a tooth that needs to be extracted, ask your dentist or implant specialist if you're a candidate for immediate loading.

WHAT IF YOU DON'T HAVE ENOUGH BONE?

There's good news for patients who previously have been told that they don't have sufficient bone for implant placement. If the surgeon, after evaluating your bone quantity and quality on x-rays or a CAT scan, believes there's not enough bone for implant placement, he or she may recommend a bone graft. A bone graft involves taking a small amount of synthetic or processed cadaver bone or your own bone from another part of your body (such as your jaw or hip) to replace lost bone elsewhere. After a period of healing, sufficient bone should be available for implant placement.

IMPLANTS AREN'T FOR EVERYONE

Dental implants aren't the right restorative choice for every patient. Poor or questionable candidates for implants include those who have:

1. Insufficient healthy jawbone to support an implant and poor prognosis for bone grafting
2. Gum disease
3. Medical conditions that affect the body's ability to heal and repair itself, such as diabetes and cancer
4. Conditions affecting the ability to use the hands and arms
5. A lack of commitment to thorough home care and professional maintenance
6. Osteoporosis that is being treated with bisphosphonates
7. A smoking habit

Orthodontics

There's no greater value in esthetic dentistry than tooth repositioning through orthodontic treatment. If you don't want to wear braces for 18 months or more, ask your general dentist or orthodontist for other options. There are almost always compromises and options available. For example, conventional braces can have either metal or porcelain brackets, and most adults opt for the porcelain or tooth-colored braces for esthetic reasons. Although this traditional approach is usually the most efficient method of repositioning teeth, there are alternatives, such as those described below.

INVISALIGN

Invisalign is one of the most popular new orthodontic methods. This technique uses a series of clear matrices that are worn over your teeth for about 20 hours a day, usually for 6 to 24 months. Each matrix moves the teeth a specific distance, then is replaced by a new matrix after 2 weeks. This process continues until the final matrix moves the teeth into the desired position. The advantage of this treatment is that no one will know you are having your teeth straightened.

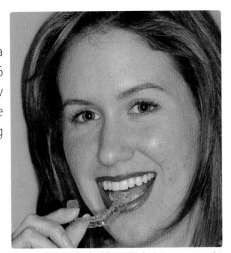

LINGUAL BRACES

Another technique to move teeth is lingual braces, which are appliances that are mounted behind the teeth and cannot be seen unless you open your mouth wide and tilt your head back or down. However, there are limited situations in which lingual braces can be used. Treatment can cost more and take longer than other techniques, and the braces may affect your speech and irritate your tongue while you're wearing them. Nevertheless, many adults who otherwise wouldn't have undergone orthodontic treatment have changed their smiles with these "hidden" appliances.

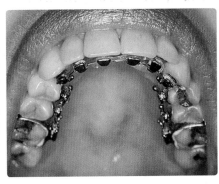

SPRING ALIGNER

A spring aligner is a removable retainer that is a good choice for someone who desires minor tooth movement in the lower incisor region but does not want braces. The aligner should be worn at least 12 hours per day, and if it is worn full-time, good results can be achieved in approximately 4 months. A spring aligner is significantly less expensive than Invisalign or lingual braces but doesn't provide as much correction.

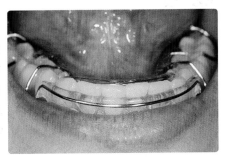

CHANGE A **SMILE**

THE PROBLEM

The high school years are a critical time in the development of a person's self-image and self-care habits. Unsightly or missing teeth invite ridicule, cause embarrassment, and can potentially seriously damage self-esteem. In addition to pain, pediatric dental disease can cause lifelong health risks, lack of confidence, and antisocial behavior, reducing a teen's ability to do well in school and, ultimately, succeed in life.

THE SOLUTION

An attractive smile restores self-esteem and improves a teen's ability to communicate without embarrassment with peers, teachers, and potential employers. It generates positive responses from others, which builds confidence and increases chances for greater success in life. In addition, it shows them the value of caring for their oral health and well-being, teaching them good habits that they can continue throughout their lifetime.

TOMORROW'S SMILES

Dr Ronald Goldstein helped found and currently chairs Tomorrow's SMILES, a special National Children's Oral Health Foundation (NCOHF) program that promotes oral health and well-being for economically disadvantaged high school students. Tomorrow's SMILES works through NCOHF's national affiliate network of nonprofit community dental facilities and volunteer private practitioners to restore students' smiles and change their lives.

BE A PART!

Please help give disadvantaged young people the opportunity to know the joys of engaging and healthy smiles. You can donate or volunteer online at www.tomorrowssmiles.org—100% of contributions go directly to teen programs.

CHANGE A **LIFE**

Tomorrow's SMILES gives disadvantaged teens a better chance for happy, successful, and productive lives.

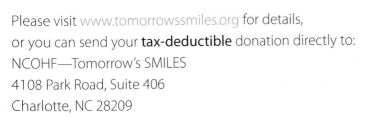

Dear Dr. Goldstein,

My name is Brittany: I am 14 years old and have a major problem with my smile. I was born with missing teeth, twelve in fact, and I am in need of help. The teeth that are in the place of my front teeth are the ones that were supposed to be beside the front teeth. They were moved closer together with braces so I could talk.

I'm not the prettiest thing you have ever seen. I'm to the point where I come home and I sit on my bed and cry because someone had called me a name and brought my self-esteem down.

I know that deep down inside that I'm not all that ugly. The people who make fun of me ask me why I haven't done anything about my problem, but all I can say is that I'm trying.

I would like nothing more than to have people smile back at me, not point and stare. All I want is my two front teeth.

Brittany

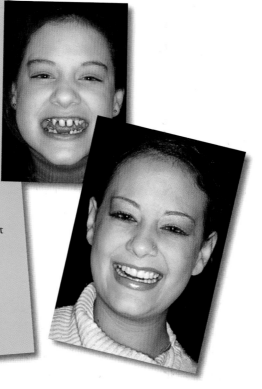

Please visit www.tomorrowssmiles.org for details, or you can send your **tax-deductible** donation directly to:
NCOHF—Tomorrow's SMILES
4108 Park Road, Suite 406
Charlotte, NC 28209

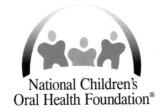

National Children's
Oral Health Foundation®

REFERENCES

No book is an island unto itself. Other works influence and spark ideas that may take other forms. If you desire additional information, consult the sources below, which constitute the major references for this book.

Bates B, Cleese J. The Human Face. New York: Dorling Kindersley, 2001.

Berns JM. Why Replace a Missing Back Tooth? Chicago: Quintessence, 1994.

Berscheid E, Walster E, Bohrnstedt G. The happy American body: A survey report. Psych Today 1973;7:119.

Caccamo R. The Right Hairstyle for Your Face Shape. TheHairStyler.com website. http://www.thehairstyler.com/the_right_hairstyle_for_your_face_shape.asp. Accessed February 20, 2009.

Christensen GJ. A Consumer's Guide to Dentistry. St Louis: Mosby, 1994.

Denholtz M, Denholtz E. The Dental Facelift. New York: Van Nostrand Reinhold, 1981.

Garfield S. Teeth, Teeth, Teeth. Beverly Hills, CA: Valient Books, 1969.

Goldstein C, Goldstein RE, Garber D. Imaging in Esthetic Dentistry. Chicago: Quintessence, 1998.

Goldstein RE. Esthetics in Dentistry, ed 2. Ontario: BC Decker, 1998.

Goldstein RE, Garber DA. Complete Dental Bleaching. Chicago: Quintessence, 1995.

Greenwall L. Bleaching Techniques in Restorative Dentistry. London: Martin Dunitz, 2001.

Haywood V. Tooth Whitening: Indications and Outcomes of Nightguard Vital Bleaching. Chicago: Quintessence, 2007.

Jablonski S. Illustrated Dictionary of Dentistry. Philadelphia: Saunders, 1982.

Kwon S, Ko S, Greenwall LH. Tooth Whitening in Esthetic Dentistry. London: Quintessence, 2009.

Liggett J. The Human Face. New York: Stein & Day, 1974.

Mechanic E. Esthetic Dentistry: A Patient's Guide. Montreal: EC Dental Solutions, 2005.

Moss SJ. Growing up Cavity Free: A Patient's Guide to Prevention. Chicago: Quintessence, 1993.

Nahai F. The Art of Aesthetic Surgery. Principles & Techniques. St. Louis: Quality Medical, 2005.

New Beauty Magazine [various issues]. 2009;5.

Patzer G. Looks: Why They Matter More Than You Ever Imagined. New York: Amacom, 2008.

Shelby DS. Anterior Restoration, Fixed Bridgework, and Esthetics. Springfield, IL: Charles C. Thomas, 1976.

Smigel I. Dental Health, Dental Beauty. New York: M Evans, 1979.

Taylor TD, Laney WR. Dental Implants: Are They for Me? Chicago: Quintessence, 1993.